A Pocket
Health Guide

Snow White

A Pocket Health Guide

LOGICAL
Publishing

LOGICAL is a publishing company registered with government organizations responsible for the development of the cultural and communications industry.

We acknowledge the support of the Canada Council for the Arts, the Department of Canadian Heritage and the Société de développement des entreprises culturelles du Québec for our publishing program.

We further acknowledge the financial support of the Government of Canada through the Book Publishing Industry Development Program for our publishing activities.

Distribution in Canada:
Hushion House Publishing Limited
36 North Line Rd., Toronto, Ontario M4B 3E2
Tel.: (416) 285-6100
Fax: (416) 285-1777
1-877-396-0777

Assistant Editor: Jacques Lalanne
Copyediting: Diana Halfpenny, Louise Carrier
Design and layout: PAGEXPRESS
Cover Design: Christian Campana
Translation: Charles Prévost

Logical Publishing
7 Bates Road
Outremont, Québec H2V 1A6
Tel.: (514) 270-0208 • Fax: (514) 270-3515
http://www.logique.com

A Pocket Health Guide

Legal deposit, 1st quarter 2001
Bibliothèque nationale du Québec
National Library of Canada

ISBN: 1-895919-67-3
LPX-041

Printed in Canada

Contents

. . . .

Part One

Nutrition
and Health

Foreword

. . . .

This book is intended as a guide for anyone who wishes to improve his health by learning more about choosing and combining foods, so as to facilitate digestion and the assimilation of nutrients and the elimination of toxins.

With the help of specific guidelines, the reader will be able to evaluate his state of health and track its changes, through the symptoms he observes in his own body, and thus gain a better understanding of its strengths and weaknesses.

It has been shown that, with age, we become increasingly vulnerable and less energetic. The bad habits acquired over the years gradually diminish our immune system's effectiveness and adversely affect our nervous system.

Our metabolism then becomes less sensitive and it loses its ability to regulate body functions. To regain balance and energy, we must first start with courage and determination, and then take a few minutes every day to observe the changes in our state of health, so as to understand and improve the factors that have been neglected.

It is imperative that we accept the importance of good health habits, especially as regards a balanced and evolving diet. According to epidemiological studies, there is a higher incidence of diseases and chronic illnesses in our society. The public's general state of health is already weakened by years of harmful habits.

Numerous factors affect our health, specifically our eating habits, physical activity, rest and relaxation, emotional stability and environmental factors such as humidity, temperature variations, etc. Well-being requires a holistic approach to health.

In this book, I will be addressing two of the most relevant and important health factors with which I have worked over the years, in consultation with people who have come to me for help with their well-being: mental attitude and nutrition.

Chapter 1

STRESS AND HEALTH

O ver the past fifteen years, the incidence of numerous chronic diseases is of increasing concern for those who care about their health. Cancer has become a critical problem for modern society. The enormous amount of scientific research aimed at countering this scourge and the arsenal of medications and treatments, which are both exhausting for sufferers and expensive for society, are a burden on the national budget.

Increasingly, health specialists are promoting the concept of prevention.

Numerous studies have shown that our persistent health problems are directly related to foods saturated with chemical products and the over-consumption of animal proteins and fats.

STRESS AND THE NERVOUS SYSTEM

The central nervous system, which controls breathing, digestion, hormone levels, etc., cannot maintain a proper balance if it is placed under excessive strain.

For example: When a person hears good news, his nervous system causes him to breathe deeply, giving him large doses of oxygen and energy. The person becomes infused with joy, feels happy and is filled with internal peace. This person will then be able to eat heartily.

On the other hand, when a person receives bad news—for example, a romantic breakup, an accident or a death—his nervous system causes impaired breathing, disturbed heart beat and stiffness of the joints. His gastric functions, which are also affected, can cause inadequate digestion, stomachaches, intestinal disorders, etc., and in the long term, ulcers of the stomach or duodenum. Fear and insecurity can also trigger symptoms of physical imbalance: some will experience heat flushes while others will suffer opposite effects such as cold and shivering.

In women, fear can provoke hormonal instability, changes in the menstrual cycle and even infertility. In men, prolonged stress can lead to bladder hypersensitivity, backaches and even substantial hair loss.

Over time, a weakened nervous system can provoke severe emotional reactions—insecurity, emotional emptiness, lack of self-confidence, irrational fears, etc.—often accompanied by persistent back pain, circulation problems and stiffness of the joints. Such disturbances are not necessarily felt at the onset of internal imbalance: these health problems start surfacing after several years of accumulated abuse.

When one is young and full of energy, these problems can go unnoticed. But stress accumulated over several years, an unhealthy lifestyle, or a pessimistic outlook—often accompanied by hereditary deficiencies—inevitably lead to gradual physical degeneration.

Our automated lifestyle disregards our body's warning symptoms and leads us to compound our mistakes. After several years of neglecting our body's vain requests for rest, exercise, fresh food, clean air, pure water, etc., chronic *disease* sets in. At the root of physical deterioration one may find: psychosomatic problems (often going back to childhood), poor posture, unhealthy living conditions, noxious eating habits, digestive disorders, lack of affection, a hostile environment and the neglect of many other essential factors.

This erosion of the immune system disrupts breathing patterns, inhibits blood circulation, causes digestive or hormonal troubles, and so on. In such a devitalized organic structure, viruses and bacteria proliferate unchecked.

It is often only after decades of poor nutrition, a sedentary lifestyle, emotional damage, the breaking of family ties, lack of caring and alienation that we finally notice how weak and out of balance we have become.

When several of these elements combine, they can cause unremitting stress, which further depletes our physical energy and brings on a high risk of serious disease, including various forms of cancer.

Chapter 2
CARCINOGENS

. . . .

The terrible disease we call cancer has its origin in a variety of factors: psychic, chemical, physiological, physical and nutritional. Here are some examples.

Psychic Factors

Nervousness and psychological strain

Anxiety, emotional strain, problems with the nervous system

Unresolved family problems

Professional and work-related stresses

Mourning, depression, isolation

Sudden changes (divorce, death, unemployment, accidents, relocation, etc.)

Chemical Factors

Aflatoxin (found in peanuts)

Tar and amianthus (asbestos)

Diethyl pyrocarbonate (antiseptic ingredient added to certain fruit juices, beer and wine)

Medications (antibiotics: penicillin, streptomycin, etc.; anti-inflammatory drugs: cortisone, Aspirin; synthetic hormones, steroids, etc.), which destroy intestinal bacteria and cause digestive troubles

Antidepressants and barbiturates (sedatives and soporifics)

Aniline tinctures

Lead and mercury (leached into rivers and oceans)

Radioactive waste (dumped into the sea)

Cadmium (found in gas and water)

Strontium 90 (emitted by nuclear facilities and testing)

Nickel, cobalt (found in tobacco smoke, badly roasted coffee, etc.)

Chemicals used in agriculture (pesticides, insecticides, fertilizers)

Nitrates transformed into nitrites and then into nitrosamines (acid rain, nitrogen fertilizers, etc.)

Hormones and antibiotics (accumulated in animal meat products)

Uranium oxide (found in drinking water)

Unhealthy food combinations, toxic and acidifying foods (animal fat, sugar, refined white flour)

Consumption of toxic and non-nutritional products (sweets, coffee, alcohol, tobacco, etc.)

Food preservatives

Food additives: colorings, conditioners, anti-fungals, artificial flavorings, etc.

Chloral polyvinyl, polytetrafluorides used as anti-stick coatings on pots and pans (Teflon, etc.)

High-temperature cooking (pressure cooking)

Over-heated oils and fried foods (as in Chinese cooking, for example)

Etc.

Physiological Factors

Stomach ulcers

Congenital malformations

Intestinal problems

Hormone problems (some symptoms: painful menstrual cycle, heavy menstrual flow, headaches, nervousness, swollen belly, painful armpit ganglia prior to period, cysts in breasts during ovulation)

Vaginal tract infections

Physical Factors

Classic electrotherapy: electrical current, ionization, etc.

Electromagnetic radiation in all frequencies and repeated exposure: ultrasounds, mammograms, etc.

Magnetic fields, for example hydro-electric fields located too close to residential areas, cell phones, etc.

Radioactivity: exposure to a radioactive source, such as X-rays, for example

Removal of beauty marks

TYPES OF CANCER AND POSSIBLE CAUSES

Thanks to epidemiological and nutritional research, the influence of nutrition on health is better understood. We know now that regular consumption of certain products is tied to the incidence of several diseases, specifically cancer.

Cancer of the esophagus

➤ More common from 40 to 50 years of age

Drinks and foods that burn the esophagus (very hot tea or water)

Overeating, especially before going to bed

Meals eaten too fast

Insufficient mastication of solid or raw foods

Alcohol and fermented drinks

Ingestion of mouldy bread or rice

Cancer of the esophagus is frequent in Japan, mostly in men, who drink very hot tea.

Cancer of the esophagus is prevalent in the populations of tropical and temperate regions.

Consumption of alcohol raises the percentage of cases in certain European and Asian countries.

Stomach cancer

➤ More common from 35 to 64 years of age

High-fat diet

Monosodium glutamate

Mustard, nutmeg, pepper and curry

Smoked meats and fish

Cooking with heavy oils

Stress

Stomach cancer is common in Chile, where many fried and hot spicy foods are eaten, and in Japan, due to the heavy use of monosodium glutamate.

Colon cancer

➤ More common from 35 to 64 years of age

Diet containing too much meat, fat and smoked fish

Food coloring and artificial flavors

Canned goods

Beer

Strong spices (mustard, pepper, curry, etc.)

Work-related stress

Difficult social and economic situation

Colon cancer is more prevalent in Europe, particularly in Scotland, in the Americas and in Africa.

Brain cancer

➤ More common from 6 to 40 years of age

Air pollution and lack of oxygen

Chemical preservatives in foods

Canned goods

Radioactivity (high-voltage electric lines, television)

Dairy products, especially cheeses from cows' milk containing traces of herbicides

Prepared meats

Sweets, chocolate

Stress

Exposure to computers without protective screens

Exposure to cell phones

Brain cancer is common in North America.

Cancer of the liver

➤ More common from 30 to 40 years of age

White rice

Peanuts and commercial peanut butter

Yellow coloring in margarine (paradimethyl-amino-azobenzene)

Diethyl-pyrocarbonate, used as an antiseptic in beer, wine and certain fruit juices

Alcohol

Fungicides

Meat fried in butter

Cancer of the liver is common in Asia and central Africa.

Lung cancer

➤ More common from 45 to 55 years of age

Tobacco

Amianthus mine pollution (asbestos)

Pollution from aluminum production

Air pollution: cadmium and other substances emanating from automobile gasoline

Stale air in buildings, especially during winter

Radioactivity

Lung cancer is common in North America. It can be aggravated by the cold and by poor nutrition.

Breast cancer

➤ More common from 35 to 50 years of age

Hormone problems. Symptoms: inflammation of the uterus, mammary cysts

Heredity

Consumption of animal fat

Prolonged use of estrogens and progesterone

Coffee, alcohol, chocolate

Obesity

Making love every day does not make you sick... on the contrary!

Breast cancer is very common in North America, due to high consumption of meat, sugar, cheese and pastries.

Cancer of the larynx

➤ More common from 30 to 60 years of age

Tobacco

Alcohol

Poor oral hygiene

Anemia

Cancer of the larynx is common among smokers and those who consume large amounts of sugar.

Thyroid cancer

➤ More common from 40 to 60 years of age

Thyroid-related hormone problems

Iodine deficiency

Digestive problems

Anemia

Thyroid cancer is very common among women who live in cold countries, due in part to a lack of sunlight.

Cancer of the lymphatic system

➤ More common from 20 to 30 years of age

Tobacco

Meat and fat consumption

Anemia

Stress

Cancer of the lymphatic system is very common in North America.

Bone cancer

➤ More common from 10 to 25 years of age

Consumption of animal fat

Excessive exercise

Unbalanced diet in certain athletes

Fluoride

Skin cancer

➤ More common from 25 to 50 years of age

Prolonged exposure to the sun

Arsenic and lubricating oil pollution

Radioactivity

Cancer of the bladder

➤ More common from 40 to 50 years of age

Beer

Contact with certain chemical substances, specifically aniline

Chronic urinary tract infection

Tobacco

Prolonged contact with paint, shoe polish, etc.

Cancer of the bladder is very common in taxi and truck drivers, people who work standing up, on railways, in radio and television stations, in laundromats or the gasoline industry.

Cancer of the pancreas

➤ More common from 40 to 45 years of age

Animal fat

Alcohol

Food containing chemical additives

Kidney cancer

➤ More common in 40-year-old men

Meat and organs

Salt and sugar

Kidney cancer occurs mostly in the United States, in Canada and in France.

Testicular cancer

➤ More common in 20- to 40-year-old men

Hormone imbalance

Testicular blockage from birth

Uterine cancer

➤ More common in 40- to 55-year-old women

Pre- and post-menstrual hormone problems

Constipation or chronic diarrhea

Recurring vaginal infections

Prolonged use of estrogens and progesterone

Estrogens and growth hormones used in the meat industry (chicken, lamb and beef)

Coffee, alcohol

Sweets, chocolate, ice cream, pastries, etc.

Dairy products

Uterine cancer is prevalent in North America. Fatty foods and stress are major factors.

Prostate cancer

➤ More common from 48 to 60 years of age

Meat

Alcohol and coffee

Chronic urinary tract infection

Kidney trouble

Hormone problems

Prostate cancer is very common in North America.

Cancer of the mouth and oral cavity

➤ More common from 40 to 50 years of age

Tobacco

Alcohol

Chewing tobacco

Betel nut chewing

Cancer of the mouth and oral cavity is very common in Asia, particularly among women.

Leukemia

➤ More common from 6 to 45 years of age

Anemia

Radioactive products, specifically strontium 90

Sweets: chocolate, candy, pastries

Leukemia occurs in young anemic children and in pre-menopausal women.

PREVENTIVE MEDICAL EXAM

A preventive medical examination will put your mind at rest. At a certain age, it is a good idea to start having regular check-ups. If specific symptoms occur, a more detailed examination will provide better insight into your condition.

The sooner signs of health imbalance are detected, the sooner we can act to correct them. Here are certain signs you should be alert for.

For men and women

Starting at 35 years of age, have a yearly medical check-up. Those who smoke and drink alcohol, hot chocolate or hot tea should have a mouth cavity examination. See your doctor if you have any of the following symptoms:

- Digestive problems (repeated bouts of diarrhea, chronic constipation, stomachaches before or after every meal)
- Frequent vomiting during or after meals
- Weight or appetite loss
- Sudden difficulty breathing
- Persistent backache, accompanied by coughing
- Persistent headache accompanied by vision problems
- Dizziness accompanied by headache
- Blood in the stool or permanent rectal pain
- If frequent sexual relations with multiple partners are the norm

For women

Starting at 45 years of age, see your doctor if you have any of the following symptoms:

- Abnormal warming of the breasts before, during or after menstruation
- Painful and heavy menstruation
- Recurring vaginal infections
- Unusual lumps in the breasts

Between 48 and 55 years of age, see your doctor if you have any of the following symptoms:

- Abundant and prolonged menstruation (10 to 12 days)
- Insomnia
- Heat flushes
- Skin disorders
- Nervousness and anxiety, fatigue, irritability, quick loss of temper, impatience, highly emotional state
- Poor digestion, flatulence

From 45 years on, see your doctor if you have any of the following symptoms:

- Excessive abdominal pain with cramps and vaginal discharge, especially of a yellowish or greenish color (risk of cyst and tumor formation)
- Unusual breast symptoms
- Unusually developed and painful beauty marks (never attempt to remove beauty marks yourself)

For men

From 45 years on, see your doctor if you have any of the following symptoms:

- Problems while urinating
- Blood in the urine

Chapter 3

MENTAL ATTITUDE AND HEALING

CANCER AT DIFFERENT AGES

The mind and the spirit play an important role in healing. The hypothalamus transfers our emotional reactions to the pituitary gland and influences hormonal balance. The power of the body's natural defenses is strongly influenced by our emotional state, the quality of our personal relations and our will to live. In many cases, these factors have made all the difference!

The will to heal and the quality of one's energy allow the body's natural defenses to give better protection against abnormal cells.

Whether in a child, an adolescent or an adult, high stress levels, poor nutrition, an unhealthy environment, a sedentary lifestyle and a negative psychosomatic attitude can cause unbalance, which will become manifest sooner or later as pains and *dis-ease.*

In children and adolescents, the effect of the will to live on health and healing is crucial. Children are sometimes more vulnerable than adults to harmful environmental influences.

TELLING TESTIMONIALS

Here are a few case histories of people suffering from different ailments that I have met over the years.

———

Gilbert, who suffered from brain cancer, wanted to change his diet in order to regain his health. At first, he showed strong will because his girlfriend supported his efforts; they were in love and wanted to get married as soon as he got better. With my help, his nutrition improved over a two-year period. His health improved and stabilized. His doctors confirmed this progress.

Some time later, he resumed his old eating habits (cakes, sweets, ice cream, meat, soft drinks, wine and coffee), stopped exercising and lost his *joie-de-vivre*. Two years later, I learned that he had had a relapse: he suffered from headaches, frequent dizzy spells, etc.

———

Gérald, an athletic 55-year-old full of energy, who played golf every weekend and spent his winter holiday in Florida, discovered he had lung cancer.

Upon learning of his disease, he decided to retire and radically change his lifestyle. I realized how determined he was to get better when he asked me to help him define a personalized diet. Vitamins, tonics and herbal teas replaced coffee, tobacco and sweets. His health improved rapidly. After two years of these new habits, he now considers himself saved, and plays golf with his friends with a restored sense of well-being.

Cancer can strike at any age. Healing depends on the individual: on his thoughts and his ability to heal. In such situations, parents can help their children adopt a constructive attitude and improve their lifestyle.

———◆———

Jeanine, 45, was afflicted with polycythemia, for which she had undergone repeated chemotherapy treatments. Much weakened—her complexion was pale, her hair dry and brittle, her eyes wan—she wanted advice about her diet and what vitamins would reinforce her immune system. She was very patient and showed a great deal of resolve in trying to cure her health problems by all possible means. Supported by the love and care of her husband and children, she managed to regain her health. Five years later, she wrote to me:

> "From our very first meeting, you restored my confidence and my hope for a better life. The balanced diet you recommended, the vitamin supplements and other suggestions that you gave changed my life in a matter of weeks. I noticed a dramatic improvement in my state of health: all the ailments that used to trouble me have subsided and finally disappeared almost completely. You helped me regain the necessary strength and motivation to recover my health. I want to tell you how grateful I am for all your care, support and wisdom."

———◆———

Rolland, 42, had kidney cancer. He'd already had one kidney surgically removed and one year later, metastases were found in his other kidney.

He came to me, hoping that I could help him recover his health, since no other regular treatment could help him. After changing his lifestyle and especially his diet according to my recommendations for one year, it was found that he had no more metastases.

He then wrote me:

> "I want to thank you for your advice regarding nutrition and vitamins; with your diet, I have recovered my health. I'm writing not only to thank you, but to let those who consult you know that they can trust you, and to exhort them never to lose hope. Your regimen is very strict, but it is really worthwhile."

———◆———

Eric, a six-year-old boy, suffered from brain cancer. Since birth, this child drank milk, ate buttered white bread, candy, chocolate and cheese every day. He refused to start eating whole wheat bread, whole rice or other grains. He would eat no vegetables.

His parents asked me to prepare a diet designed to improve his health, but they were not convinced of its effectiveness and so failed to insist that the child follow it.

His immune system grew daily weaker and, sadly, he died.

———◆———

Unbalanced nutrition seems to be a given in most children suffering from brain cancer. Their digestive system is affected by constipation or diarrhea. They frequently suffer from headaches, which naturally affects their disposition.

⟹•⟸

Benoît, a 15-year-old adolescent, also had brain cancer. His parents came to me for help. When I asked him if he wanted to live, he answered unhesitatingly "Yes!" He then gathered his strength to confront the disease. Because he really wanted to live, I could make him understand that he had to listen to his mother and eat the food she prepared for him, because a healthy diet would help him beat the cancer. Loved and supported by his parents, brothers, sisters and an aunt, this teenager was able to improve his lifestyle, starting with his diet. I recommended fresh juices, fruit, organic vegetables, grains, Soya, tonic and vitamins.

After three months, he was able to leave the house for daily walks, helped by his mother. After eight months he returned to school, and in spite of a two-year hiatus because of the disease, he was able to resume his schooling at the same level as his peers.

He wrote me these words:

> "Let me tell you, this disease really messed up my adolescence on the physical level. But, thanks to the diet you prescribed, I was able to beat it. I'm 23 now; I can enjoy the simple pleasures of life, and I hope to maintain the innocence that won out over my analytical nature and helped me overcome this obstacle. I want to take this opportunity to extend my heartfelt thanks for all your help, that enabled my parents and me to beat my sickness. You contributed to this victory and I am very grateful."

41

Benoît is now 25 years old and attending university. He still maintains the same diet that we implemented during his teenage years. His health is a wonderful example of deep healing. In spite of his youth, he had resolved to heal and improve his lifestyle to attain that goal.

—⇒◆⇐—

In all these cases, as in many others, the road to recovery starts with a positive attitude and the determination to change one's lifestyle. The sooner we overcome psychological problems that can hinder healing, the faster we recover our health. In children and adolescents, the will to live is often powerful and healing possibilities are strong. At any age, a fundamental change in lifestyle is required—nutrition, level of activity, rest, behavior, and attitude—as well as traveling the long road to wisdom and, often, recovery.

Psychological factors

When an imbalance is detected in weak or ailing people, most of the time they have been suffering from digestive difficulties for a long time. They have a poor diet and their food combinations make digestion difficult. Whether they eat a lot or a little, they digest hardly any of what they consume. Their challenge is then to re-create a healthier, more well-balanced lifestyle.

People in poor health show signs of nervous tension—exteriorized in outgoing people, held inside in introverts—that is often related to issues such as breakup, financial failure or the loss of a loved one.

In such situations, the person must act quickly and keep up the improvements to his lifestyle. If he is supported by family and friends, in spite of his weakened state, he will have the energy he needs to recover, even from the brink of death. This improvement takes place gradually and will last for the rest of his life.

The strength of the will to live varies from one person to another. But obsessive preoccupation with one's state of health can lead to mental anguish and pain.

Calmness, insight into the origin of our pain and problems, the affection and encouragement of loved ones, the hope of improving our condition, active visualization of our progress and trust and confidence in our chosen health counselors improve our chances of healing.

The decision to alter one's lifestyle entails a long-term commitment. It's not a question of following some diet for a while and then resuming old habits, but rather of radically transforming one's way of life. Often, this change is more successful if implemented gradually, as the knowledge and understanding of one's metabolism progressively consolidate and clarify the decision. To succeed, this way of living must conform to our ideas and grow in a climate of trust and awareness. Our health will improve through patience, will and discipline.

Informed optimism is essential when one is faced with disease, especially with what we call "cancer"—we think we are doomed, especially if we have undergone treatment, which has exhausted our reserves of mental energy. If the problem is compounded by loss of family or work, separation from our partner or loved ones, or other such difficulties, we then become very vulnerable. Anxiety, isolation, worry and fear increase stress levels. We then often forget about our capacity for healing and recovery, as well as our powerful propensity for life.

Obviously, such beliefs profoundly affect our morale. This emotional suffering is often more painful than anything else. If a person convinces himself that he has no chance of healing, the despair and depression that follow can lead to total collapse of the immune system. This stress and insecurity can unbalance the suprarenal glands, which are essential in eliminating free radicals and other toxins from the tissues.

Although our condition requires immediate attention and carefully chosen and administered care, the decision to live and a confident attitude remain essential factors in recovering vital energy and strength.

During my 30 years of experience in epidemiological research and then as a nutritional advisor, I have noticed that most people whose health is unbalanced are physically exhausted and psychologically discouraged.

Some display signs of energy and a strong will to live; these people still entertain positive thoughts about their health. Those surrounded by family and affectionate people whom they can count on, who feel loved, nurtured and cared for, have more positive thoughts and can clearly visualize their progress. Their state of health improves rapidly.

On the other hand, those who feel abandoned by or isolated from family and friends, who lack affection or suffer financial insecurity, heal more slowly and are much more prone to relapses.

Even if they want to improve their lifestyle based on the suggestions of a professional, they get discouraged if they feel alone, especially if their new way of life isolates them from the rest of their family. They give up their new regimen for lack of encouragement and energy.

Thanks to a positive psychological attitude, a change in lifestyle, and in particular the adoption of a new diet, many who were considered incurable have considerably improved their state of health in just a few months. Unfortunately, as soon as they consider themselves healed, some resume their old habits and return to the same torpid state.

The vitality of the immune system must be supported by an appropriate lifestyle.

RELAPSE

In my practice, I have noticed that patients treated by conventional means who do not improve their diet and other habits have relapses, often within two years of treatment.

The letdown they feel is then very strong and their energy is depleted; because of this weakened mental state, crippling anxieties can then set in and take over. In my experience, this relapse is often merely the result of an accumulation of toxins.

The treatments they received have caused a weakening of the immune system. Medication irritates the digestive tract, especially the intestines, and often causes loss of appetite and a decrease in energy. Chemotherapy destroys cancerous cells, but also diminishes white blood cell count and generally weakens one's state of health.

We also have to build up the strength of the digestive system. If it has been worn out by 10, 20, 30, 40 or 50 years of abuse and has been forced to operate at maximum capacity, we will have to let it rest and regenerate.

A healthy diet, rich in vegetable proteins and in vitamins and minerals, is vital in improving our health. To regenerate our cells it is important to make immediate and permanent changes to our eating habits.

As we have seen, the psychological factor is crucial to maintaining and recovering health. To tap into this important aspect of healing, there are a number of proven techniques that people can try out and practice, based on what suits them best.

A FEW HEALTH-ENHANCING PSYCHOLOGICAL TECHNIQUES

Visualization

➤ To attain a specific goal, it is essential to visualize. For example, we must imagine our health improving, our energy being regenerated. We must picture ourselves exercising, accomplishing tasks, meeting people, etc. All these thoughts can help dissipate anxiety and insecurity.

➤ Thought control, meditation, yoga and T'ai Chi are all ways to relax and free the mind from useless tension.

➤ Every person, no matter what his talents and inclinations, can write poetry or make music in rhythm and harmony with nature, to free his soul from anything that might burden it. We can:

– Write or draw about what bothers us;

– Sing our own words to music we have made up;

– Cultivate peace in our life;

– Create a different life for the future.

Appreciation of Nature

➤ Our state of health improves when we immerse ourselves in the love of nature.

➤ As we walk through a forest or in the mountains, we can appreciate trees, birds and animals, breezes, running water, etc.

Cultivating Energy-Enhancing Relationships

➤ Creating a more romantic love life warms the heart.

➤ Travel and different surroundings make us more adaptable.

➤ Making new acquaintances, establishing sincere relationships, going out with new friends are an important part of a full life and full recovery.

➤ Always learning and finding out new things stimulates us and keeps us young.

➤ Whether our talents are great or small, making music, singing and playing for relaxation, drawing, painting or writing create constructive channels for our energies.

Preserving our Inner Child

➤ Having fun horsing around, marveling at the sight of a butterfly or the sound of a bird, rediscovering activities we enjoyed in our youth are all good ways to cultivate our energy and make it flow.

➤ If you have a pet, experience the peace of playing with it outside.

Keeping Busy

➤ Tinkering with and inventing things, working with our hands (making furniture for example), cultivating a garden or cooking constructively occupy body, mind and spirit and keep anxiety from invading our thoughts.

➤ Volunteer work helps us forget our own problems by caring for and helping others.

➤ Spending time with children, playing with them, talking and listening to them, drawing or making music in their company keeps us in touch with their vitality and *joie-de-vivre.*

➤ Taking part in social activities, playing chess, dancing, going to friendly gatherings, etc., promotes physical, psychic and emotional well-being.

➤ Going to happy, joyful places, where children or adolescents are having fun, keeps our sense of wonder alive.

➤ Outdoor activity and exercise, boating, bicycling, volleyball, walks in the woods, golf or any other sport maintain a positive mental attitude.

➤ Some form of outdoor activity or exercise, twice daily, is a must at any age!

CULTIVATING DAYDREAMS OR WAKING DREAMS

Daydreams can be an escape, a way of liberating the spirit. Through daydreams, we can accomplish the following:

➤ Conjure up people we have loved in the past or love in the present; relive the joy or pleasure we felt in their company;

➤ Express our feelings of pain, our anger at those who have been hurtful to us in the past. To regain our peace of mind, we must choose to forget the pain and forgive those who caused it;

➤ Cry alone or better still, on the sympathetic shoulder of someone we love, for this allows us to relinquish hate and disappointment that have kept us, sometimes since childhood, from realizing our full potential;

➤ Laugh a lot… for the time that is allotted to us is short;

➤ Write down important memories, from early childhood right through our lives until today and tomorrow;

➤ Become conscious of the psychological difficulties caused by ill health;

➤ Review life's good and bad moments;

➤ Talk about our glory days, our happy times, etc.

Take care of the nervous system

➤ Don't give bad news to sick people.

➤ Avoid emotions that can affect the nervous system.

➤ Avoid watching television for too long.

➤ If you are sick, don't spend hours on the telephone.

➤ Don't worry about petty things.

➤ Avoid sadness and anger.

Rest

➤ The spirit needs calm.

➤ The body needs relaxation.

➤ Massage is excellent for removing toxins from the body and regulating blood circulation.

➤ Relaxation through meditation and Chi Gung exercises is extremely effective, for the spirit cleanses the being of fatigue and stress.

➤ When the mind is clear, digestion is improved and concentration and decision-making skills are sharper.

Through these various techniques, a person becomes his own therapist and creates his own placebo effect.

Chapter 4
FOODS AND THEIR PROPERTIES

A healthy diet requires a majority of alkalinizing foods. Acidifying foods lead to fatigue and vulnerability to infections.

ALKALINIZING, ACIDIFYING AND NEUTRAL FOODS

Fruits and vegetables are alkalinizing.

Butter and vegetable oil are neutral.

Grains, beans, seeds and nuts are acidifying.

Dairy products, meat and seafood are very acidifying.

Fruits

Fruit is an excellent source of vitamins and minerals whose natural sugars are easy to digest.

They make great snacks. They are best eaten fresh and in season, and if possible tree-ripened; this is when they contain the most vitamin C and natural sugars and are therefore easiest to digest.

The following list of foods contains a breakdown of their elements and properties.

Apples

➤ Vitamins C, A

➤ Potassium, silica, magnesium

➤ Pectin

➤ Help digestion in the intestine

➤ Ease pain in the joints

➤ Decrease nervous tension

Apricots

➤ Vitamins A, B, C, PP

➤ Rich in magnesium, potassium, iron, calcium, sodium, sulfur, manganese, fluoride, cobalt

➤ Sugar

Avocado

➤ Non-saturated fat

➤ Calories (200 cal/100 gr)

➤ Cystine, tryptophane, tyrosine

➤ Liposoluble vitamins A, E, PP

➤ Rich in calcium, sodium, magnesium, and especially potassium (beneficial to the nervous system)

Bananas

➤ Vitamins A, B1, B2, C and E

➤ Phosphorus, magnesium, potassium, iron, zinc, sodium

➤ Sugar

➤ Pectin

➤ Easily digested when tree-ripened and eaten alone

Bananas, dried

➤ Sugar

➤ Calories (300 cal/100 gr)

➤ Phosphorus, calcium

➤ Vitamins B1, B2, C and PP

Lemons

➤ Vitamins A, C, PP, B1 and B2

➤ Promote fixing of calcium and other minerals

Melons (cantaloupe, yellow melon, honeydew melon and watermelon)

➤ Vitamins A, C, B1

➤ Phosphorus, calcium and iron

Oranges

➤ Vitamins C and PP

➤ Calcium, phosphorus, magnesium, sodium, iron, copper, zinc

➤ Help formation of teeth and tendons

➤ Strengthen blood vessels and cellular exchanges

➤ When tree-ripened, constitute an active antioxidant and assist in cancer prevention

Papaya

➤ Vitamins A, B1, B2, C and D

➤ Easily digested, helps maintain intestinal balance

Persimmons

➤ Vitamin A

➤ Sugar

➤ Easy to digest

Pineapple

➤ Calories (50 cal/100 gr)

➤ Sugar

➤ Vitamins B1, B2, B6, PP and C

➤ Iodine, manganese, iron, potassium, calcium, sulfur, magnesium, zinc and copper

Vegetables

Certain vegetables, such as Brussels sprouts, spinach, chard and eggplant, contain harmful substances, such as oxalic acid. This is why it is better to consume them steam-cooked so as to neutralize this acid, and limit their daily consumption.

Cabbages are better digested if eaten raw or as sauerkraut (naturally fermented and containing lactic acid).

Artichokes

➤ Stimulate liver function

Beets

➤ Rich in minerals

Broccoli, cauliflower

➤ Best eaten raw, to prevent fermentation

Burdock

➤ Promotes bladder and kidney functions

➤ Encourages regeneration of damaged tissue

➤ Contributes to resistance against skin infections

Carrots

➤ Fortify the liver

➤ Increase production of red blood cells

➤ Rich in vitamin A and good for eyesight

Celery

➤ Helps eliminate water in the tissues

Cucumber

➤ Rich in potassium

➤ Contributes to skin regeneration

Dandelions

➤ Contain vitamins A and C

➤ Rich in potassium, iron, manganese and chlorophyll

➤ Diuretic

➤ Help reduce blood cholesterol levels

Note: Eat the leaves and drink the tea made from the roots

Eggplant

➤ Gently stimulates the liver and activates pancreatic secretions

➤ Helps get rid of intestinal worms

Escarole

➤ Rich in potassium

➤ To be eaten raw or taken as tea

➤ Assists kidney function

Garlic

➤ Stimulant, diuretic and expectorant

➤ Regulates blood pressure

➤ Helps reduce blood cholesterol levels

➤ Encourages elimination of harmful bacteria

➤ Reduces respiratory infections

➤ Should be eaten raw

Green beans

➤ Low in sodium

➤ Promote liver and pancreas functions

Leeks

➤ Contain vitamins C and B

➤ Rich in iron, magnesium, sulfur, silica, potassium, manganese and calcium

➤ Diuretic

Lettuce

➤ Rich in potassium

➤ Has a calming effect

Mushrooms

➤ Rich in potassium, phosphorus, silica, magnesium, calcium, sulfur

➤ Contain amino acids and polysaccharides

➤ Strengthen the immune system and overall vitality

Onions

➤ Contain vitamin C

➤ Rich in potassium, phosphorus and carbohydrate

➤ Stimulant, diuretic, scurvy preventive, aphrodisiac

➤ Promote proper kidney function

➤ Encourage sleep

➤ Assist weight loss

Peppers

➤ Contain vitamin K, P and chlorophyll

➤ Strengthen blood vessels

➤ Stimulate gastric secretions

Plants and roots

➤ Burdock root, Indian rhubarb, sorrel, watercress, seaweed, knapweed and red clover (Essiac extract) are renowned for their diuretic and antioxidant properties.

Pumpkin, squash

➤ Contains vitamin A

➤ Rich in potassium

➤ Promotes concentration and memory

Radishes, black

➤ Stimulate bile production by the liver

➤ Reduce respiratory and kidney troubles

➤ To be taken as an infusion or as a syrup

Radishes, red

➤ Contain potassium

➤ Stimulate the respiratory tract

Spinach, chard

➤ Rich in iron, potassium, folic acid and oxalic acid

➤ Contributes to cell repair

➤ Boosts red blood cell production

Turnip

➤ Contains potassium

➤ Promotes respiratory system function

➤ Contributes to the reduction of pulmonary irritations

Watercress

➤ Contains vitamin A, carotene, B1, B2, C and PP

➤ Rich in potassium

➤ Contributes to red blood cell production

Herbs

Cinnamon

➤ Stimulates digestion

Fennel (seeds)

➤ Enhances proper activity of the digestive system

➤ Facilitates liver function

➤ Helps dissolve excess fat

➤ Increases maternal milk production during breastfeeding

Licorice

➤ Helps soothe stomach and intestinal cramps

➤ Gentle laxative

➤ Helps regulate low blood pressure

➤ Helps reduce menstrual problems

➤ Promotes female fertility

➤ Heightens pulmonary activity

Mint

➤ Stimulates the appetite and helps digestion

➤ Reduces digestive gasses

➤ Stimulates the intestine and freshens the breath

Mugwort

➤ Helps eliminate gasses

➤ Helps regulate the menstrual cycle

➤ Combats kidney inflammation

Parsley

➤ Contains vitamins A and C

➤ Stimulates kidneys and bladder

➤ Very effective at reducing kidney stones

Plantain (leaves)

➤ Diuretic

➤ Encourages blood coagulation

➤ Promotes fertility

➤ Settles diarrhea and soothes hemorrhoids

Rue (leaves)

➤ Strengthens the uterus

➤ Has antiseptic properties

➤ Helps protect the body against infections

Sage

➤ Stimulates the appetite

➤ Has a calming effect

➤ Promotes liver and kidney functions

➤ Regulates menstrual problems

Tarragon

➤ Promotes memory and brain activity

➤ Strengthens the liver

Beans

Chickpeas

➤ Contain vitamins B and C

➤ Help drain the urinary tract

Peas

➢ Rich in vitamin C

➢ Contain iron and phosphorus

➢ Contain fiber that stimulates the digestive tract

Nuts

Nuts are rich in protein, fats and carbohydrates, and contain vitamins B and E.

Almonds

➢ Contain vitamins from the B group

➢ Rich in phosphorus, potassium, calcium and magnesium

➢ Calories (600 cal/100 gr)

➢ The easiest nut to digest

Seeds

Seeds are rich in protein, vitamins A, B, E and fats.

Pumpkin

➢ Rich in iron and phosphorus

➢ Calories (550 cal/100 gr)

➢ Help control urinary infections

➢ Reduce prostate inflammation

Sesame

➤ Calories (563 cal/100 gr)

➤ Rich in potassium, calcium, iron, magnesium, chrome, copper, silica

➤ Called "the longevity food" in Asia

➤ Improve endocrine balance

➤ Contribute to the development of the brain and the nervous system

Sunflower

➤ Rich in iron, potassium, calcium, phosphorus, copper

➤ Calories (570 cal/100 gr)

➤ Help reduce cholesterol buildup in the bloodstream

➤ Promote stomach activity

SOME FOOD TRANSFORMATION METHODS

Lacto-fermentation

Fermentation produces lactic acid. Fermented vegetables containing lactic acid are easier to digest and assimilate. They help regulate intestinal activity. Their fermentation makes them predigested and reduces the work of intestinal bacteria. In addition, they help produce vitamins as they pass through the intestine.

Sprouting

Sprouting increases the vitamin and enzyme content in seeds. It retains the fiber and minerals which help digestion.

Starches are thus converted into simple sugars, proteins into amino acids, fats into fatty acids, and are more easily assimilated. Sprouted seeds contain a lot of chlorophyll. They supply easily assimilated minerals.

Among others the following seeds can be sprouted: alfalfa, clover, sunflower, buckwheat, mung bean, chickpeas, fenugreek and radish.

Grass Juice

Wheat grass and barley grass contain 70% chlorophyll and are a great source of calcium, iron, magnesium, phosphorus, sulfur, cobalt, zinc, vitamins C and A and choline. Because of their alkalinity, these grasses help oxygenate the blood.

These cereal grasses can be eaten as is or, more often, dried and powdered, or yet again liquefied through a juice extractor.

Wheat or barley grass and alfalfa, clover, radish and fenugreek sprouted seeds contain from 30% to 70% chlorophyll.

Sprouted wheat, oat, rye, buckwheat and bean seeds contain from 5% to 10% chlorophyll.

Chapter 5
FOOD PREPARATION METHODS

Proper food preparation is essential to preserving its nutritional value, freshness and digestibility.

WASHING

Wash vegetables quickly, without letting them soak for long periods in water.

COOKING

Cooking in water significantly reduces vitamin content; for example, cooking can destroy 40% of vitamin C.

This loss can be minimized by keeping the peel on the vegetables and cooking them in very little water.

Steam or pressure-cooking prevents vitamins from dissolving in the water.

Liposoluble vitamins (A, D, E, K) remain stable when exposed to heat and will not dissolve in cooking water.

Cook foods in ceramic, stainless steel, Pyrex or enamel cast-iron cookware. Food cooked in aluminum pots becomes contaminated through oxidation.

OXIDATION

The effect of heat: Heat accelerates oxidation of vitamin C. The longer the cooking time, the greater the oxidation.

A higher temperature and shorter cooking period reduces the loss of nutrients.

To limit the loss of hydro-soluble vitamins (B, C) through oxidation, reduce cooking time, cook foods whole and cook vegetables in an environment which is neither too acid nor too alkaline, quickly, at high heat. (*Note:* An alternate method of avoiding oxidation is to steam vegetables slowly, at very low heat.)

Vitamin loss through oxidation is greater during dry heat cooking (in the oven), where temperature rises more slowly.

The effect of cold: cold prevents oxidation of vitamin C.

The effects of oxidases: oxidases are destroyed by heat.

Practical Hints

➤ Store foods in a cold place

➤ Buy food fresh and consume within a short time

➤ Avoid adding sodium bicarbonate to cooking water

➤ Limit cooking time for vegetables so they are *al dente,* as the Italians say ("crunchy to the tooth")

➤ Avoid reheating food

Raw Food

➤ Use stainless steel graters

➤ Use ceramic or porcelain jars and pots

Preserving Vitamin Content

➤ Vitamin A is not affected by heat, but oxidizes upon contact with air

➤ The B vitamins are quite resistant to oxidation, although vitamin B2 will be destroyed if exposed to light, especially in an alkaline environment

➤ Vitamin C is very fragile and oxidizes easily if exposed to light or heat

Preservation of oils

➤ Oils oxidize easily. It is better neither to overheat them nor to use them in frying

➤ They are better preserved cold, in the dark and protected from drafts

Eating for nourishment

➤ Steam vegetables slowly or blanch them in water for three minutes

➤ Eat four or five small meals a day

➤ Avoid large meals, especially at night

➢ Wait two hours before having dessert

➢ Avoid drinking during meals

➢ Eat slowly, in peace and quiet

➢ Avoid strong emotions (anxiety, bad moods, etc.) during meals

➢ Try and prevent constipation or diarrhea

Vitamin Loss

Many factors can cause vitamin loss in foods. Specifically:

➢ Preparation or cooking methods

➢ Factors augmenting dissolving, oxidation and changes due to light

Chapter 6
A HEALTHY DIET

Maintaining a proper diet remains a complex issue. Many factors influence our system's ability to assimilate nutrients. Here are a few essential, tried and true rules that will help improve your health and vitality.

HEALTHY FOODS

Consume a significant quantity of foods containing:

➤ Dietary fiber

➤ Antioxidant vitamins A, C, E

➤ Easily-absorbed minerals

These elements are plentiful in fresh and raw fruits and vegetables, and in whole grains.

In particular, try to eat the following:

➤ Dark fruits and vegetables

– Apricot, cantaloupe, peach, etc.

– Spinach, tomato, red pepper, etc.

➤ Cruciferous vegetables

– Cabbage, broccoli, Brussels sprouts, etc.

➤ Vegetable proteins

– Legumes, Soya, nuts, almonds, etc.

Use quick and simple cooking methods. Avoid large, complicated meals.

➤ Do not consume alcoholic beverages or soft drinks to excess.

Avoid

➤ Stimulants: coffee, black tea, chocolate

➤ Spicy foods

➤ Foods containing artificial coloring or flavors

➤ Greasy sauces

➤ Excessive fat (too much cheese, butter, milk)

➤ Sweets (candy, pastries, soft drinks, etc.)

Other healthy habits

➤ Walk barefoot over grass, earth and rocks, to maintain the body's electric balance. Grass, for example, gives off oxygen ions that ionize the air and promote activity as well as a sense of calm and relaxation.

➤ Avoid exposure to the sun's rays without skin protection. This is especially true for fair-haired women, whose skin is more sensitive.

FOODS ESSENTIAL TO THE IMMUNE SYSTEM

Choose fruit, vegetables and nuts that are in season. All
must be fresh and preferably organically grown.

Fruit (in season)

Apples
Apricots
Bananas
Barbary figs
Blueberries
Cantaloupe
Cherries
Cranberries
Dates
Durians
Figs
Grapefruits
Grapes (black, blue, red, green)
Ground cherries
Guavas
Kiwis
Lemons

Limes
Melon
Nectarines
Oranges
Papayas
Peaches
Pears
Persimmons
Pineapples
Plums
Pomegranates
Quince
Raspberries
Strawberries
Tangerines
Watermelon

Vegetables (in season)

Artichokes	Jerusalem artichokes
Asparagus	Leeks
Beets	Mushrooms: reishi, shi-
Bell peppers, red and green*	itake
Broccoli*	Okra
Burdock	Onions
Cabbage, green or red (raw)	Parsnips
Carrots	Potatoes
Cauliflower*	Pumpkins, all kinds
Celery	Radishes: black, red
Celery-root	Rappini
Chinese cucumbers	Sauerkraut
Convolvulus	Spinach
Eggplant*	Squash
Endive	Sweet potatoes (yam)
Garlic, raw	Tomatoes, ripe
Ginger	Turnip
Green beans	Zucchini*

Grasses

Wheat grass, barley grass

---

* To be eaten raw or semi-cooked to avoid fermentation in the digestive tract.

Vegetables (leafy)

Basil
Bok choy
Chard, green
Chard, red
Celery
Chicory
Chives
Citronella
Collard greens
Coriander (cilantro)
Dandelion
Escarole
Fennel
Fines-herbes, fresh
Green onion

Lambs' lettuce
Lettuce: Chinese, romaine, curly
Marjoram
Mint
Nappa
Parsley
Rosemary
Sage
Spinach
Tarragon
Thyme
Watercress
Wild thyme
Young plantain

Sprouts

Alfalfa
Bean
Buckwheat
Clover
Lentil

Mung
Radish
Soya
Sunflower
Etc.

Beans

Adzuki
Black-eyed peas
Chickpeas
Lentil
Lima

Mung
Red beans
Soya
White beans

Note: Eaten in moderate quantities and properly combined with other foods, beans will not cause flatulence.

Tofu

Tempeh and tofu

Note: Dried tofu is less acidic and easier to digest.

Whole grains

Arrow-root	Pearl barley
Buckwheat	Quinoa
Corn	Rice (sweet, or brown)
Millet	Rye
Oat	Wheat

Note: Most of the above grains can be eaten as a broth with a pinch of sea salt, according to taste.

Whole seeds

Fenugreek	Pumpkin
Linseed	Sesame (black, brown, white)
Melon	Sunflower
Psyllium	

Pasta (once in a while)

Buckwheat	Soya
Quinoa	Wheat
Rice	

Note: Whole-wheat noodles are definitely more nutritious.

Bread

Buckwheat	Rice
Kamut	Rye
Millet	Spelt
Multi-grain	Wheat

Note: Sourdough and sprouted-seed breads are more easy to digest, although it may take a while for the digestive tract to get used to them.

Pastries

One may occasionally eat homemade cakes or cookies (without salt, fat, eggs, or commercial baking powder).

Raw nuts

Almonds	Pecans
Brazil nuts	Pine nuts
Cashew nuts	Walnuts
Hazelnuts	

Note: It is better to eat no more than five nuts a day. Preferably, buy nuts in their shells.

Nut butter

Almond	Sesame
Cashew	Sunflower
Hazelnut	Tahini
Lecithin	

Seaweed

Arame	Kombu
Dulse	Mekabu
Hijiki	Nori
Kelp	Wakame

Drinks

Almond milk	Lotus root (powdered)
Amazake	Mu 9
Bancha tea	Mu 16
Herb tea	Rice milk
Kudzu	Soya milk
Kukisha tea	

Seasonings

Fines-herbes

Gomashio (sesame, seaweed and sea salt, ground and lightly roasted)

Kombu (seaweed)

Light tamari

Salt-free powdered vegetables

Tekka (miso, Soya, vegetable roots)

Teriyaki

Umeboshi (medicinal plums)

Vegetable salt

Oils

Olive, saffron, sesame, sunflower, Soya, peanut, corn, safflower, pumpkin, grape seed, linseed, hazelnut, walnut, canola.

Note: First cold-pressed oils are definitely more nutritious and less harmful. Do not consume more than two tablespoonfuls daily.

Sauces

Barley miso, brown rice miso (light or concentrated)

Note: Miso is made from fermented Soya, barley or rice with salt and water. To be consumed in moderate amounts.

Dairy products

Cheese (white skim)
Goat's milk (*Note:* Organic goat's milk is preferable, as it is more easy to digest.)
Kephir
Skim milk
Whey
Yogurt

Fresh eggs

Eggs from grain-fed hens are definitely more nutritious. Do not exceed three eggs a week.

Note: Poached or soft-boiled eggs are most nutritious.

Fish, poultry and lean meat

Carp	Lamb	Sole
Chicken	Ostrich	Trout
Cod	Partridge	Turbot
Cornish hen	Pheasant	Turkey
Goat	Pike, yellow or walleyed	Veal
Grouper	Quail	
Haddock	Rabbit	

Note: Animals raised and fed naturally are nutritionally far superior. Boiling, poaching, grilling and other no-fat cooking methods help retain nutrients.

Sugars

Rice syrup, malt powder, natural honey, stevia, blackstrap molasses.

Note: Choose non-pasteurized products.

Salt

Gray sea-salt   Seaweed salt   Vegetable salt

Herb teas

Boldo   Dandelion   Saint John's wort
Burdock   Juniper   Sarsaparilla
Centaury   Red clover

Note: Using one teaspoon of an equal-part mix of all these herbs, steeped in three cups of water, makes an excellent cleansing and purifying tea.

Fruit or vegetable juices

The juices of fruits and vegetables that are in season provide us with nutrients that are easily assimilated.

Grass juices are rich in vitamins A, B and C, in chlorophyll and active enzymes.

For example, have 125 ml to 250 ml (4 to 8 oz) of half juice, half water for a morning snack.

In the afternoon, drink a glass of vegetable juice, preferably lacto-fermented.

Fresh juices made in a juicer, *without added sugar or salt*, are definitely more nutritious.

Fruits

Apples	Grapes	Papaya
Black currants	Honeydew melon	Plums
Cherries	Melon	Quince

An example of a fruit juice cocktail:

Apple juice + pear juice + half water

Vegetables

Beets	Carrots	Potatoes (raw)
Cabbage (raw)	Celery	

One may mix several vegetables in the same juice. Here are some examples of vegetable juice cocktails:

Cucumber (¼) + celery (2 stalks) + parsley (6 sprigs) + half water

Carrots (2) + celery (2 stalks) + parsley (6 sprigs) + half water

Beets + celery + parsley

Cucumber + celery + parsley

Broccoli + celery + parsley

Use *distilled or spring water* rather than tap water, which contains chlorine and often also fluoride and harmful metals.

EXAMPLES OF MEALS AND SNACKS

Upon rising

Juice from naturally-ripened fruit

or wheat grass juice

1 hour later: Breakfast

Grains or bread and sesame butter

Tonic

Vitamins

Herb tea

10 o'clock: Snack

A piece of fruit

or fruit juice

or Soya milk

or rice milk

or goat's milk

or skim milk

Ginseng

or royal jelly

Whole grain broth

Noon: Light lunch

Steam-cooked vegetables

Whole grains (rice, millet, quinoa, etc.) with sesame

or fish, boiled, grilled or poached

or lean meat (no meat if one is sick)

Salad with seeds or seaweed

Herb tea

Vitamins

3 or 4 o'clock: Snack

Bread and goat's cheese, *or* sesame butter, *or* vegetable pâté

or goat's milk yogurt with blackstrap molasses and nuts

or rice cake with applesauce or whole grain broth

or sushi

or homemade cake

or fruit pudding

or sweet potato

or sweet rice with sesame

Tonic

Herb tea

5 o'clock

Vegetable juice

or raw vegetables (carrot and/or celery and/or cucumber)

6 o'clock: Light meal

Vegetable soup
Whole grains
Beans *or* tofu *or* fish
Steam-cooked vegetables
Salad with seaweed
Herb tea
Vitamins

8 or 9 o'clock: Snack

Herb tea
Bread with sesame, almond or sunflower butter
or sugar-free cookie
or royal jelly
or one piece of fresh fruit, or fresh fruit compote
or tonic
or whole grain broth

Vitamins and natural supplements
(to be taken with meals)

Vitamin A (beta-carotene)
Vitamin B complex or active brewer's yeast
Vitamin C
Fish liver oil
Vitamin E
Minerals

Bone meal or calcium lactate

Calcium with magnesium and vitamin D3

Kelp

Digestive enzymes for people over 50

or multivitamins and minerals

Lifestyle choices

➤ Keep temperature in the house between 18 °C and 20 °C

➤ Maintain relative humidity between 30% and 50%

➤ Sleep with the window slightly or wide open, depending on the season

➤ Take a 15 to 30 minute nap in the afternoon

➤ Do physical exercise outdoors every day: walking, jogging, bicycling, cross-country skiing

➤ Take a walk after the evening meal

➤ Breathe deeply several times a day in a park or on a mountain

➤ Do relaxation exercises: yoga, meditation, gentle gymnastics, T'ai Chi

➤ Do a dry scalp massage at least once a day

➤ Take one or two massages a month (Swedish, Californian, shiatsu, Chinese, etc.), especially during the winter, to improve circulation and resistance to the cold

➤ Take two or three baths a week

➤ Add to the bath water:

    ¼ cup of Dead Sea salt

    1 tablespoon of sweet almond oil

Avoid

➤ Stimulants, for they irritate mouth and digestive tract and destroy vitamins B and C:

Alcohol	Refined sugar
Coffee	Chocolate
Black tea	Monosodium glutamate (MSG)

➤ Tobacco

Avoid foods that cause fermentation

Acidic vegetables:	Rhubarb, tomatoes
Butter:	Peanut butter
Canned goods:	All canned foods
Cold cuts:	Any kind of sliced meats
Condiments:	Vinegar, ketchup, salad dressings, oriental sauces: oyster, mushroom, or hot sauce
Dairy products:	Milk and cheese from hormone-treated cows, cooked butter, strong cheese, 15% to 35% cream
Drinks:	All kinds of soft drinks
Eggs:	From hormone-fed chickens
Fried foods:	Any kind of fried food
Fruits:	Dried fruit with sulfites

Meats:	Beef and pork, meat from hormone-treated animals, smoked meat or fish
Oil:	All refined oils
Pastries:	Commercial pastry—cake, cookies, pie, pizza
Preservatives:	All foods containing preservatives and artificial coloring
Refined flours:	White bread, pasta, white noodles
Refined grains:	Couscous, white rice, white wheat flour
Salt:	Refined white salt
Sauces:	Mayonnaise
Seafood:	Shrimp, lobster, crab, scallops, mussels, clams, anchovies
Snacks:	Ice cream, chewing gum, candy
Spices:	Pepper, nutmeg, mustard, curry
Sweets:	White sugar, syrups made from refined sugars

Vegetables prone to vitamin A and C loss through cooking cause fermentation and should be eaten in moderation: cauliflower, broccoli, eggplant—blanch quickly (2 or 3 minutes) in hot water and eat half-cooked. Vegetables then retain their color.

FOOD COMBINATIONS

Certain foods can be easily combined and will then be properly digested. Other combinations are not good and will be difficult to digest.

For example, an apple and a pear combine well, but an orange and rice do not.

Very Easy Fruit Combinations

When we eat only one kind of food at a time, and if the food is light, then digestion is very easy.

Examples:

Eat a melon

or three apples

or a bunch of fresh, ripe grapes

There are three kinds of fruits: Acidic, semi-acidic and non-acidic (neutral).

Combining the same kinds of fruit ensures easy digestion. Fruits, especially combined according to their acidity levels, are very easy to digest, when ingested alone. Wrongly combined foods place a strain on the digestive system and cause acidity, bloating and gas.

Examples of proper combinations:

➤ Acidic fruits: Mangoes, apricots, strawberries, kiwis, oranges and raspberries

➤ Semi-acidic fruits: Pears, grapefruits, pineapples, grapes, plums, blueberries, dates, fresh figs

➤ Neutral or non-acidic fruits: Melons, papayas, apples and bananas

Easy Combinations

Vegetables can be easily combined with grains and fats *or* with protein. (Combining grains and protein makes digestion difficult.)

Examples:

Grains and vegetables

➤ Sourdough bread: rye, millet or rice, etc., with sesame or almond butter

Protein and vegetables

➤ Chicken and celery, carrot, leek and *Fines-herbes*, raw garlic and parsley

➤ Tofu and asparagus, endive, zucchini, with parsley and Soya sauce

➤ Boiled egg with spinach, green beans, etc.

➤ Rice cake or sprouted bread, artichoke and olive oil with lime juice

➤ Fish and carrots, onion, fennel, etc., and *Fines-herbes*

Difficult Combinations

Combining "sweet" vegetables with acidic ones makes digestion difficult.

Examples:

Sweet potatoes, carrots, turnips, potatoes and tomatoes, eggplant

Combining grain or protein with sweet foods makes digestion very difficult and often causes flatulence.

Examples:

Pancakes and fruit or maple syrup

Baked beans: beans + lard + maple syrup

Omelet + maple syrup

Bread and jam or honey or maple syrup

Combining protein (especially animal protein), such as meat and cheese for example, with grains and certain vegetables, especially acidic ones, makes digestion very difficult.

Examples:

Meat and potato, tomato, onion and eggplant

All-dressed pizza: white dough + meat + vegetables + tomato + cheese

Spaghetti with meat sauce: pasta + meat + tomato + peppers + cheese

Quiche: wheat flour + eggs + melted cheese + ham + spinach + tomato

Examples of highly improper combinations:

Cereal + protein (milk, for example) + sugar + fruit

Bread + orange juice + eggs + bacon + coffee + sugar or hot chocolate

MASTICATION

Proper digestion starts in the mouth, so it is essential to chew each mouthful 10 to 30 times. If one is in a hurry, it is preferable to eat several small meals throughout the day.

Chapter 7
VITAMINS AND MINERALS

Vitamins are complex organic substances contained in minute amounts in foods. The human body does not itself produce vitamins. It extracts these essential elements from the foods we consume. Deficiencies of vitamins and minerals have a negative effect on body functions.

The vitamins locked in foods are fragile and can be damaged or destroyed by preservation methods, heat, cooking and drying.

VITAMINS

The main vitamins and their uses

Vitamin A

➤ Ensures quality of mucus membranes

➤ Helps to protect the body against infections

➤ Protects against the damage caused by air pollution

➤ Improves blood quality in the capillaries by contributing to a better oxygenation of tissues

➤ Is an important cancer-preventing antioxidant

Natural sources

Vegetable

Beets and other colored vegetables
Cabbage
Carrots
Dandelion
Dark green, leafy vegetables

Pumpkin
Spinach
Tomatoes
Turnip

Colored fruit

Apricots, oranges, peaches, plums

Animal

Butter, milk, cream, fatty cheese, egg yolk, fish liver

Vitamin B complex (B1, B2, B3, B5, B6, B12, biotin, choline, inositol, folic acid, paba)

➤ Necessary in the formation of red blood cells and nerves

➤ Promotes digestion of carbohydrates

➤ Essential elements in the formation of carbohydrates

➤ Builds up resistance to infections

Natural sources

Vegetable

Almonds	Lentils	Rye
Bran from whole grains	Millet	Sesame
Brown rice	Nuts	Soya
Corn	Oats	Sunflower
Grains, legumes	Peanuts, roasted	Wheat
Green beans	Peas	

Brewer's yeast contains large amounts of the B complex group.

Animal

Fish, chicken, eggs, liver, beef, lamb, pork

Choline (from the B group):

➤ Helps to digest, absorb and carry lipids and liposoluble vitamins (A, D, E and K) to the bloodstream

➤ Reduces metabolic fat

➤ Is necessary for the synthesis of nucleic acid, DNA and RNA

➤ Regulates and improves liver and bile function

Natural sources

Vegetable
Soya, wheat germ, Soya lecithin

Animal
Egg yolk

Vitamin C (ascorbic acid)

➤ Antioxidant, helps prevent cancer

➤ Essential to glandular function

➤ Helps prevent infections

➤ Ensures quality of gum tissues and teeth

➤ Prevents physical and mental exhaustion

➤ Helps counteract the effects of environmental and air pollution

➤ Regulates gastrointestinal disorders

➤ Stimulates the appetite

➤ Raises energy levels

➤ Promotes scar-tissue healing

Natural sources

Vegetable

All fruits and vegetables, such as:

Apples	Broccoli
Black currants	Cabbage
Cherries	Cabbage leaves
Durians	Dandelions
Guavas	Green peppers
Limes	Parsley
Oranges	Potatoes
Persimmons	Spinach
Pomegranates	Tomatoes
Rosehips	Turnip
Strawberries	Turnip leaves

Ester C

This C vitamin with neutral pH (non-acidifying) is made up of mega-molecules from several ascorbates, specifically from naturally chelated calcium ascorbate, which allows for better absorption.

Vitamin E

➢ Antioxidant, helps prevent cancer

➢ Enhances blood circulation and cardiac endurance

➢ Enlarges blood vessels and improves circulation

➢ Essential to sexual organ function and fertility

Natural sources

Vegetable

Cold-pressed oils, wheat germ oil, Soya oil, nuts, seeds

Animal

Eggs

Vitamin F (linoleic acid)

➤ Regulates glandular activity, especially of the suprarenal glands

➤ Contributes to calcium and phosphorus availability for the cells

Natural sources

Vegetable

Cold-pressed oils:
Corn, linseed, safflower, saffron, Soya, sunflower

MINERALS

A number of minerals are necessary to vital body functions. The main ones are listed below.

Calcium

Functions

➤ Essential to the formation of bones and teeth

➤ Essential to muscle contraction

➤ Necessary for blood coagulation

➤ Contributes to the activity of many enzymes

➤ Helps maintain sodium-potassium-magnesium balance

➤ Essential for efficient use of phosphorus and vitamins A, C and D

Natural sources

Vegetable

Almonds
Broccoli
Brussels sprouts
Cabbage
Dandelions
Lettuce
Nuts

Red chard
Seeds
Sesame
Sunflower
Vegetables, dark-colored, raw
Walnuts
Watercress

Animal

Milk and cheese

Magnesium

➢ In combination with calcium, essential for cardiovascular endurance

➢ Essential for building teeth and bones

➢ Promotes absorption of other minerals such as calcium, phosphorus, sodium and potassium

➢ Promotes scar-tissue healing

Natural sources

Vegetable

Alfalfa	Dried fruit	Red chard
Almonds	Figs	Sesame
Apples	Kale	Soya beans
Beet leaves	Limes	Sunflower seeds
Cabbage	Nuts	Vegetables, dark-green
Celery	Peaches	Whole grains

Phosphorus

➢ In combination with calcium, essential for building bones and teeth

➢ Important for metabolizing carbohydrates

➢ Essential for maintaining acid/alkaline balance in the blood and tissues

Natural sources

Vegetable

Whole grains, seeds, nuts, vegetables, dried fruit, corn

Animal

Dairy products, egg yolk, fish

Iodine

Essential for thyroid gland function

Natural sources

Vegetable

Acidic fruits, pineapples, pears
Chard, green turnips
Seaweed, kelp, dulse
Watercress, artichokes, garlic

Animal

Fish liver, egg yolk

Selenium

➤ Antioxidant whose properties are akin to those of vitamin E

➤ Protects blood cells from oxidation damage

Natural sources

Vegetable

Brewer's yeast, kelp, garlic, grains, vegetables

Animal

Milk, eggs

VITAMIN AND MINERAL SUPPLEMENTS

Goat's milk whey

Goat's milk whey is a derivative of dehydrated goat's milk. This concentrated alkaline food contains very little protein, which makes it very easy to assimilate.

➤ It increases intestinal flora.

➤ It can relieve stomachaches and constipation.

Acidophilus

Acidophilus contains more than eight billion living bacteria per gram: *lactobacillus acidophilus, lactobacillus casei var, rhamnosus, lactobacillus bifidus, streptococcus fæcium.*

Bacteria living in the colon are important to the proper functioning of the gastrointestinal system and promote absorption of nutrients through the colon walls for use by the body. They represent at least 30% of fecal mass.

These bacteria strengthen the immune system. They produce certain B complex vitamins, for example vitamin

B12. The lactic acid they produce improves digestion and nutrient use. Through the production of lactic acid and bactericides, intestinal flora reduces pathogenic bacteria.

Shark cartilage

Shark cartilage contains proteins and minerals, specifically calcium, phosphorus and carbohydrates: all substances which stimulate the immune system and act as a metabolic nutriment.

Shark cartilage has been administered with positive results to people suffering from such ailments as: skin diseases, degeneration of the retina, arthritis and inflammation of the joints.

Shark oil

This medium-chain fatty acid extracted from shark livers has immunogenic properties. It contains practically no cholesterol.

Also:

➢ It promotes healing

➢ It relieves respiratory tract irritation

➢ It speeds up recovery following pneumonia or other infections

➢ It promotes formation of antibodies, lymphocytes and white blood cells in the blood

Chapter 8
MY HEALTH-VITALITY TONIC

· ·

HOW MY TONIC CAME ABOUT

Having left the warm temperature of my homeland in 1967, I had to adapt to a much harsher climate, as well as an occidental diet high in animal protein. This type of nutrition seemed my best bet for withstanding the winter cold. But after adopting this new diet, I noticed that my health was deteriorating steadily. I had many colds; I often felt tired and unable to concentrate. I became more and more irritable and my energy for all kinds of activities decreased. I developed a cyst the size of a pea on my shoulder. All this gave me food for thought.

I returned to my previous way of eating, and the cyst disappeared. At that period, my diet was even more important as I was pregnant with my first child. I went looking for foods from different countries that were very high in nutritious vegetable proteins. With these I created a mix, which I called "my tonic."

My daughter was born in the middle of winter, in superb health. After breastfeeding her for five months, I also started giving her my tonic mix, adapted for infants. I observed her calm disposition and long sleeping hours.

She would spend most of her day outside, well bundled up in her baby carriage, and was thus very early on acclimatized to cold weather and temperature changes. Her complexion was clear, her cheeks naturally rosy and her eyes bright. Due to the oxygen she breathed every day as well as to her healthy diet, she was full of energy and had fine mental abilities.

I fed my two other children in this manner and was very happy with the results.

Thanks to a healthy diet during pregnancy and to proper feeding of their babies after birth, a great number of mothers who have consulted me have had healthy infants who have grown well, without tears or colic, or any of those problems that we take for granted as part of early childhood. Subsequently, these children performed well at school.

After being interviewed on television in 1982 by Jacques Boulanger, I was astounded to receive numerous requests for my tonic from all across Canada and from Vermont.

Four years later, during a TV show, the actress Andrée Boucher talked about the effectiveness of "the Snow White tonic" in combating "the November doldrums." I received so many requests—I still get emotional when I think about it—and felt so enthused by public reaction to my methods that I started trying to find ways to adapt my tonic to the many needs that had been expressed and submitted.

As a result of these efforts, I have produced this tonic for those who came to me for help in improving their health, and they have reaped the benefits: their energy has increased, their immune system is stronger and their resistance to seasonal temperature changes has improved, especially in winter. My tonic has been just as effective in increasing the strength of athletes as it has been in improving the concentration of intellectuals.

I have since been consulted by people suffering from a variety of ills, such as hypoglycemia, asthma, ulcers, etc. Each required a particular kind of care and different precautions as to the makeup of the tonic. I have therefore created several formulas, specifically adapted to various afflictions, that seem to produce excellent results.

I often hear complaints about the taste of the tonic: "It's terrible, it's so bland!" I have even been asked to change its composition to improve the flavor. Each time, I have to explain that I dare not risk reducing its effectiveness and that one just has to get used to the taste! You will find that its benefits are well worth it. (When diluted in a small glass of fruit juice, I actually find it quite tasty.)

This tonic is an extremely potent energy food, easy to prepare and practical for traveling.

During a trip to Asia in 1987 I was worried about catching tropical diseases so I brought along a good supply of tonic and vitamins for breakfast. This was a big help in my travels from one city to another. What's more, I didn't have to worry about getting sick in places where I thought the food might have been prepared under unhygienic conditions. Thus I avoided the fate of my fellow travelers, who suffered from too much heat, and from fever and indigestion.

Every morning, even if I'm in a hurry, I never miss taking my health-vitality tonic. I have found that it gives me energy and resistance to fatigue. It also helps me avoid mid-afternoon munchies, as I take it twice a day.

The excellent results obtained by hundreds of people encourage me to keep spreading the word about its effectiveness.

THE INGREDIENTS IN SNOW WHITE'S TONIC

I have created a concentrated tonic of vegetable proteins, vitamins and minerals. It is to be taken every morning, in addition to vitamin C, acidophilus and calcium.

Soya	*Contains:*	Whole proteins (comparable to animal protein). Easily digested.
	Function:	Builds muscles, strengthens the nervous system, stimulates estrogen production.
Lecithin (complex Soya lipids)	*Contains:*	Phosphorus, present in the nervous system and in cell membranes.
	Function:	Helps reduce cholesterol build-up in blood.
Rice bran	*Contains:*	Protein. Fiber. B complex vitamins (B1, B2, B3, B5 and B6).
	Function:	Nourishes the nervous system, kidneys, and intestine. Tones muscle and hair follicles.
Wheat germ	*Contains:*	Vitamin E. Protein. Non-saturated fats. Linoleic acid.

	Function:	Improves blood circulation. Tones heart and arteries. Renews skin cells.
Brewer's yeast	*Contains:*	B complex vitamins, including B12. Minerals (zinc, iron, chromium, selenium).
	Function:	Helps digestion of starches. Nourishes hair follicles. Increases maternal milk production. Helps prevent breast cancer.
Malt powder	*Contains:*	Barley protein. Sugar.
	Function:	The liver and pancreas store the proteins and sugar and release them slowly into the bloodstream.
Barley grass	*Contains:*	B complex vitamins. Vitamin C. Chlorophyll. Fiber.
	Function:	Strengthens the immune system. Helps the intestine eliminate toxins. Delivers oxygen to the tissues.
Spirulina (freshwater algae)	*Contains:*	Complete proteins. Vitamin B12. Minerals.

109

		Iron, potassium, phosphorus. Chlorophyll.
	Function:	Strengthens the immune system. Helps maintain energy. Builds resistance to infections. Nourishes hair follicles.
Kombu (sea weed)	*Contains:*	Vitamins A, B, C, D, E, K. Iodine. Proteins.
	Function:	Helps fortify glandular systems. Helps strengthen the nervous system.
Flower pollen	*Contains:*	Proteins. Essential and non-essential amino acids.
	Function:	Natural antihistamine. Fortifies glands, in particular the sexual glands.

MY HEALTH-VITALITY TONIC RECIPE

Mix these ingredients thoroughly in a blender.

6 tablespoons Soya protein
3 tablespoons lecithin
3 tablespoons rice bran
2 tablespoons wheat germ
1 tablespoon brewer's yeast †
1 tablespoon malt powder †

½ teaspoon barley grass
½ teaspoon spirulina
½ teaspoon Kombu seaweed
¼ teaspoon flower pollen †*

Store in the refrigerator.

Dilute one teaspoon of this mix in a glass of fruit juice (*organic* apple, grape or papaya).

Breakfast tonic

1 teaspoon of tonic (the quantity of tonic can be increased *slowly*, up to 2 *tablespoons*)
¼ teaspoon calcium ascorbate crystals (vitamin C)
¼ teaspoon acidophilus

I drink this tonic at breakfast, but it can also be taken 2 or 3 times a day. For children and seniors, add calcium, magnesium and lecithin.

For people suffering from constipation, add goat's milk whey (fresh or powdered) and barley grass juice.

---

† People suffering from *Candida albicans* should take the tonic without the pollen, yeast or malt.
* People suffering from gastric or intestinal problems, or who are allergic to pollen, should take the tonic without pollen.

Chapter 9
FASTS AND CURES

By eating less and resting more, the body uses less energy for digestion and muscular activity and more for elimination and tissue restoration.

Fasts and cures are ideal methods for encouraging this elimination process.

FASTING

Fasting is an effective way of eliminating toxins from the body. A great many people have cured themselves by fasting from 7 to 21 days, or even longer.

Fasting under the professional supervision of someone proficient with this technique is strongly recommended.

During a fast, we must avoid being alone or expending undue energy. We must also suspend taking medication or following medical treatment.

Fasting consists of total rest and ingesting only water and certain vitamins and minerals. This process requires supervision and special care.

After a fast, we resume eating gradually, by taking only juices for one or two days, then eating raw fruits and vegetables for three or four days, etc.

CURES

A cure consists of light eating, taking juices, fruits and vegetables, from three to 21 days.

For centuries, cures using either grapes, apples, figs or melons have been used with success.

The grape cure and the carrot juice cure (using half fruit and half water) yield good results and promote restoration of the stomach and intestine.

Following a cure, one progressively increases the quantity of food eaten. Here are a few examples of menus, which are to be adapted to the subject's condition and constitution.

TYPICAL POST-JUICE CURE MENU

7 or 8 o'clock	Wheat grass juice and lukewarm water Fruit juice and water Fruit
10 o'clock	Melon juice and water *or* papaya and water Tonic made from proteins, grains and vitamins
Noon	Fresh vegetable broth Grain broth: barley, oat, wheat, brown rice, millet and sesame (see recipes) *or* green vegetable purée

or rice or millet with sesame
Salad with sesame, sunflower and pump-
kin seeds (chew 30 to 50 times)
Herb tea and vitamins

3 or 4 o'clock   Vegetable juice (carrot or cucumber and water)
or protein and grain tonic

6 o'clock   Fresh vegetable broth
or barley broth
Salad and seaweed *or* green vegetable purée
Millet and sesame
Herb tea and vitamins

8 o'clock   Oat or barley broth

When we fast or follow a cure, we must take vitamins and supplements, specifically vitamins A, B, C, E, and natural minerals (calcium and magnesium), because they help rebuild the immune system.

Part Two

Snow White's Recipes

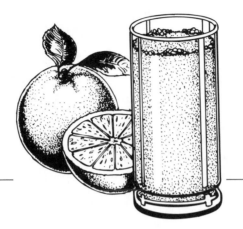

Juices

Morning Juice

Apple	Black currant*	Pear and plum
Apple and pear	Grape	Pineapple*
Apricot	Grapefruit*	Wheat grass
Barley grass	Orange*	

Beneficial mix for the gall bladder:
Juice of half a lime and olive oil (1 tsp.) mixed in a glass of lukewarm water

Mid-Morning Juice (10 o'clock snack): Fruit Juice

Honeydew melon
Papaya and watermelon, in equal parts

Afternoon Juice: Vegetable Juice

Examples
2 carrots
or a quarter cucumber
2 celery stalks, 6 parsley sprigs and water

---

* People who are sensitive to certain foods are better off not eating these fruits.

Fruit or Vegetable Juices

(Preferably lacto-fermented)
Carrot, beet, celery
From a juicer (juice must be made without added sugar or salt), maximum one 4 to 8oz glass a day, <u>half-juice, half-water</u>: Grape, cherry, plum, pomegranate, black currant, <u>watermelon</u>, quince, celery, raw potato, <u>carrot</u>, cranberry, beet, papaya, raw cabbage

Cucumber Juice

Cucumber + celery + parsley + water

Broccoli Juice

Broccoli + celery + parsley + water

Carrot or Beet Juice

Carrot or beet + celery + parsley + water

Watermelon Juice

(Red + white flesh) + water

Turnip Juice

Turnip + celery + parsley + water

Dandelion Leaf or Burdock Root Juice

A piece of burdock or ¼ cup dandelion leaves + celery + carrot + water

Wheat Grass or Barley Grass Juice

(A container of fresh or frozen wheat grass or barley grass juice + 2 oz distilled water)
Apple juice + pear + water
Papaya juice + water

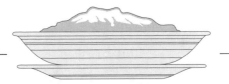

Breakfast
Grains

Porridge

1. Cook oatmeal in water

2. Add sesame or sunflower seeds to taste

3. Serve with Soya milk or rice milk

Oat Bran

1. Cook at low heat for 10 minutes

2. Serve with Soya milk or rice milk
   2 cups spring water *or* distilled water
   or ¼ cup oat bran
   or ¼ cup powdered barley
   ¼ cup brown rice flour

Granola

Granola is a mix of various grains and nuts and is sold in health food stores.

To be eaten <u>without</u> sugar *or* <u>with</u> malt, if preferred
It can be served with rice milk *or* Soya milk*

---

* People with digestion problems are better off avoiding Soya milk with their grains, because it may cause gas and flatulence.

Mixed-Grain Cereal

1. Mix 3, 4, 5, 6, 8, 12, 14 or 15 different types of grain
Example: Oats and wheat, barley, millet, rice, rye, linseed
and buckwheat

**2. Cook for 30 minutes (or 5 to 10 minutes if grains have
been soaking overnight)**
2 cups distilled *or* spring water
½ cup grains

3. Mix with nuts, seeds (sesame, sunflower, pumpkin)
or dried apples, if desired

Note: Do not add sugar, milk or other fruit

4. Serve with rice milk

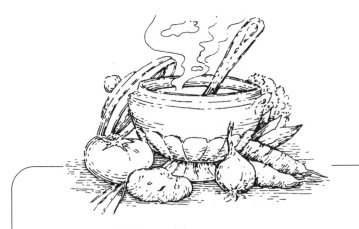

Soups
and Broths

Vegetable Broth

1. Cook for 30 minutes
2 to 3 liters distilled water
2 cups of mixed vegetables: Potatoes, carrots, celery, beet leaves, turnips, parsley and onions, etc.

2. Strain

3. Add
1 tablespoon linseeds
1 tablespoon wheat germ

4. Drink one cup of this broth (between meals)

Grain Broth

1. Cook at low heat for one hour and 30 minutes
3 liters of water
½ cup of your choice of grains: barley, black buckwheat, rye, oat, wheat, rice (according to your health objectives)

2. Drink this broth between meals

Black Bean Soup

1. Simmer on medium heat for 2 hours
   10 cups distilled water
   1 cup black beans
   ½ cup black sesame seeds
   ¼ cup adzuki beans

   Note: Add more water as needed.

2. Grind in blender

3. Strain through cheesecloth or a heavy strainer

   Note: One can also use only the water of the broth

4. Add
   ¼ cup rice syrup *or* malt

5. Serve hot or cold as an afternoon snack

Rosehip Soup

1. Heat for ten minutes
   3 cups distilled water
   3 tablespoons whole rosehips

2. Turn off heat

3. Add and mix well
   ¼ teaspoon stevia *or* 2 tablespoons malt powder
   2 tablespoons arrow-root powder

4. Serve warm as a snack

Garlic Soup

1. Cook for 5 to 10 minutes
3 cups distilled water
½ carrot thinly sliced
¼ celery stalk, thinly sliced

2. Purée

3. Serve warm

4. Add
3 to 5 cloves of finely-chopped garlic
¼ teaspoon thyme *or* oregano *or* paprika
Light Soya sauce *or* salt substitute

Raw Bean Sprout Soup

1. Mix the following in a blender:
1 cup bean sprouts
2 tablespoons soaked hijiki seaweed
2 slices crushed ginger
¼ teaspoon fennel
4 cups hot distilled water

2. Add
Light tamari sauce

3. Serve lukewarm

Sprouted Grain Soup

1. Mix the following in a blender:
3 cups hot distilled water
½ cup rye sprouts
¼ cup parsley
¼ avocado
1 tablespoon sunflower seeds
2 tablespoons light tamari sauce

2. Serve chilled

Vegetable Soup

1. Cook for 20 minutes
4 or 5 cups distilled water
¼ cup fresh lotus root, thinly sliced
½ cup carrots and celery cut in pieces

2. Add and continue cooking for another 10 minutes
1 teaspoon salt-free instant powdered vegetable broth
¼ cup wet Kombu seaweed cut in pieces
1 cup chopped watercress

3. Serve hot with rice and light tamari sauce

Chinese Vegetable Soup

1. *Cook for 20 to 30 minutes*
4 or 5 cups distilled water *or* chicken broth
½ cup soft tofu cubes *or* ¼ cup diced, grain-fed chicken
¼ cup mushrooms in pieces (white mushrooms *or* shiitake *or* reishi, soaked)

2. *Add and continue cooking for another 3 minutes*
1 to 2 cups of your choice of vegetables, cut in thin strips: Chinese cabbage, nappa, broccoli, changai, other green Chinese vegetables
1 teaspoon salt-free instant powdered vegetable broth
Light tamari sauce

3. *Serve hot with rice*

Green or Red Chard Soup

1. *Cook for 10 to 15 minutes*
4 or 5 cups distilled water *or* chicken broth
¼ cup soaked Kombu, cut in pieces
¼ cup carrot and daikon, cut in pieces

2. *Add*
3 cups green *or* red chard leaves, cut in pieces

3. *Continue cooking for another 3 minutes*

4. *Blend into a purée*

5. *Serve with light tamari sauce and rice*

Carrot and Pumpkin Soup

1. Cook for 30 minutes
4 cups distilled water
1 cup pumpkin cut in pieces
¼ cup chopped carrot
¼ cup tofu pieces

2. Add
¼ cup sliced mushrooms
¼ teaspoon *Fines-herbes*
1 green onion, cut in pieces
1 teaspoon salt-free instant powdered vegetable broth, *or* light tamari sauce

3. Serve with rice

Vegetable and Grain Soup

1. Cook for one hour
½ cup grains (rice *and/or* millet, buckwheat, quinoa, barley, etc.)
6 cups distilled water

2. Add your choice of vegetables
Carrots, celery, parsley, etc.

3. Add fish or chicken, if desired

Vegetable and Fish Soup

1. Cook for 20 minutes
4 or 5 cups distilled water
Fish: yellow pike, walleye, salmon or trout

2. Cut fish into pieces

3. Add
6 white mushrooms, cut in pieces
½ cup celery and fennel, thinly sliced

4. Cook for 3 to 5 minutes

5. Add
Green onion (*or* Italian parsley *or* fennel leaves), finely chopped
or light tamari sauce
or instant powdered vegetable broth
or fish sauce
Lime juice

6. Serve hot with rice or millet

Barley Soup

1. Cook for 50 minutes
6 or 7 cups distilled water
½ cup pearl barley

2. Add
½ carrot, thinly sliced
¼ cup celery, thinly sliced
1 teaspoon instant powdered vegetable *or* chicken broth
Light tamari sauce
Add oregano, *or* thyme, *or* paprika, *or* fennel, to taste

3. Serve hot

Rice Noodle and Lotus Root Soup

1. Cook in a tightly covered saucepan for 20 minutes
5 or 6 cups distilled water
2 slices fresh, *or* dry soaked lotus root, cut in pieces
½ cup mushrooms, cut in pieces (soaked shiitake *or* white mushrooms)
½ cup soft tofu, cut into strips
1 tablespoon salt-free instant powdered vegetable broth

2. In a bowl, put 1 or 2 cups cooked rice noodles and add
Onion, bean sprouts, coriander, green onion
Light tamari sauce

3. Serve hot

135

Lentil Soup

1. Cook for 50 minutes
6 or 7 cups distilled water
¼ cup brown *or* green lentils
¼ cup dry-roasted brown rice

2. Add and continue cooking for another 5 minutes
1 cup carrots, celery and daikon, in pieces
¼ leaf soaked Kombu seaweed, cut in pieces

3. Serve hot with
Fines-herbes, green onion, coriander, Italian parsley
Umeboshi *or* lime juice

Watercress and Tofu Soup

1. Cook for 10 to 20 minutes
4 cups water *or* chicken broth
½ cup soft tofu, cubed
¼ cup sliced white mushrooms
or 3 soaked shiitake mushrooms, sliced

2. Add
2 or 3 cups watercress
1 teaspoon instant powdered vegetable broth *or* light
tamari sauce

3. Serve with rice

Tofu and Grain Soup

1. Cook for 40 minutes to an hour
6 cups distilled water
½ cup brown rice *or* millet *or* quinoa

2. Add
½ cup soft tofu, cubed
¼ cup chopped mushrooms (soaked reishi *or* white mushrooms)
5 slices crushed ginger
½ cup sliced carrots

3. Continue cooking for another 5 minutes

4. Serve with
1 green onion cut in small pieces
1 tablespoon instant powdered vegetable or chicken broth *or* light Soya sauce *or* salt substitute

5. Add watercress or coriander, if desired

6. Add paprika or cayenne pepper, if desired

Tofu and Taro (*Colocasia*) Soup

1. Cook for 20 minutes
4 or 5 cups distilled water
1 cup peeled and cubed taro
(*or* ½ cup daikon)

2. Add and continue cooking for another 5 minutes
½ cup soft tofu, in pieces
3 chopped mushrooms (soaked reishi *or* white mushrooms)

3. Add
2 slices finely-chopped ginger
1 chopped green onion
¼ teaspoon paprika
Light Soya sauce *or* salt substitute

4. Serve hot with rice

Tofu and Spinach Soup

1. Cook for 20 minutes
4 cups distilled water
¼ cup soft tofu, cubed
2 slices fresh lotus root, finely chopped
¼ cup thinly-sliced mushrooms
(soaked shiitake *or* white mushrooms)

2. Add
1 to 2 cups Italian or Chinese spinach, chopped
1 teaspoon instant powdered vegetable or chicken broth
or light Soya sauce *or* salt substitute

3. Serve hot with rice or other grains

Rice and Chicken Soup

1. Cook for 50 minutes
6 or 7 cups distilled water *or* chicken broth
½ cup brown rice

2. Add and continue cooking for another 20 minutes
½ *or* 1 cup grain-fed chicken cut in pieces

3. Serve with
1 green onion, chopped
1 piece crushed ginger
5 to 7 sliced mushrooms
Light tamari sauce
Paprika

Rice and Veal Soup

1. Cook at low heat for 1 hour
6 cups water
½ cup dry-roasted brown rice

2. Add and simmer for another 15 minutes
½ to 1 cup ground veal

3. Serve hot with
½ teaspoon paprika *or Fines-herbes*
1 green onion, finely chopped
5 slices finely-chopped ginger
5 mushrooms, chopped
Light tamari sauce *or* fish sauce

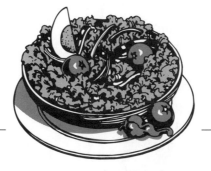

Salads

Cucumber Salad

1. Mix
1 cup sliced cucumber
½ cup roasted tofu, cut in pieces
or ½ cup roasted chicken, in pieces
¼ cup fresh mint leaves, minced
5 strips red pepper
½ celery stalk, thinly sliced
½ cup sliced carrots

2. Add salad dressing and toss

3. Garnish with
¼ cup crushed sunflower and pumpkin seeds

4. Serve with bread or rice

Chard and Cabbage Salad

1. Mix
3 cups red chard and curly leaf cabbage, chopped
¼ cup thinly-sliced onion
1 cup sprouted seeds
2 sliced white mushrooms
3 tablespoons soaked sunflower *or* sesame seeds
¼ cup cooked tofu, cut in pieces

2. Add salad dressing and toss

3. Serve with rice or cooked millet

Green Salad with Seeds

1. Mix

2 or 3 cups green lettuce leaves, chopped
¼ cup grated carrot or turnip
A bit of sauerkraut *or* ¼ cup alfalfa
1 tablespoon sesame, sunflower *or* pumpkin seeds
1 tablespoon hijiki seaweed *or* arame
¼ apple, sliced

2. Add salad dressing and toss

Vegetable and Sprout Salad

1. Mix

1 cup quinoa *or* clover *or* buckwheat sprouts
½ cup carrot
½ cucumber, grated
¼ cup chopped parsley
½ teaspoon grated ginger
½ cup chopped lettuce

2. Add salad dressing and toss

3. Serve cold on a bed of lettuce

Lacto-fermented Vegetable Salad with Seeds

1. Mix
1 cup sprouted sunflower *or* fenugreek seeds
¼ cup lacto-fermented carrot *or* beet
¼ cup chopped parsley
1 tablespoon soaked black sesame *or* pumpkin seeds

2. Add salad dressing and toss

3. Serve with rice

Tofu and Vegetable Salad with Seaweed

1. Mix
2 cups grated cabbage, carrot and turnip
½ cup cooked tofu (see tofu recipes), cut in slices
¼ cup hijiki seaweed

2. Add salad dressing and toss

3. Garnish with
Fresh mint leaves, chopped
3 tablespoons sunflower *or* sesame seeds

4. Serve with rice

Sprout Salad

1. Mix
   1 cup sunflower, buckwheat and alfalfa sprouts
   ¼ cup chopped parsley
   ¼ cup thinly-sliced apple
   ½ cup lacto-fermented vegetables

2. Add salad dressing and toss

3. Serve cold

Chickpea Salad

1. Mix
   1 cup cooked *or* sprouted chickpeas
   ¼ cup sauerkraut *or* lacto-fermented vegetables
   ½ green onion, finely chopped
   1 tablespoon soaked sunflower seeds
   ¼ cup sliced red pepper

2. Add salad dressing and toss

3. Serve cold

Rice Noodle and Tofu Salad

1. Mix

 ¼ cup roasted tofu, sliced
 ½ cup sliced carrot and turnip
 2 or 3 tablespoons crushed sunflower *or* pumpkin seeds
 ¼ cup sliced celery
 2 to 3 cups cooked rice noodles

2. Add salad dressing and toss

3. Serve cold

Salmon Salad

1. Mix

 1 thick slice steamed salmon, cut into pieces
 ¼ cup curly parsley, minced
 ¼ cup grated onion
 ½ cup mashed carrot

2. Add salad dressing and toss

3. Serve with bread or rice cakes

Tabouleh

1. Mix
1 cup pre-soaked bulgur
½ cup grated carrot
¼ cup onion, cut into small pieces
½ cup parsley, finely chopped
¼ cup cucumber, cut into small pieces

2. Add salad dressing and toss

3. Serve with bread or rice cakes

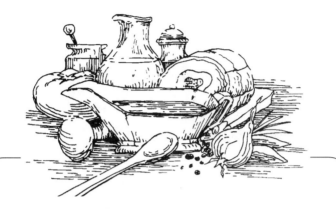

Salad Dressings

Umeboshi (concentrated plum paste)

Traditionally used to purify the blood, this sweet-and-sour-tasting marinated plum extract helps digest fats. This condiment replaces salt and vinegar in salads or on vegetables.

Oil-free Salad Dressing

1. Mix
    ¼ cup water
    2 to 3 tablespoons rice vinegar
    1 teaspoon honey
    ¼ teaspoon gray sea salt
    Lime juice, if desired

Lime-juice Dressing

1. Mix
    Soya *or* sunflower oil
    Lime juice
    Fines-herbes

2. Toss with salad

Lime and Tahini Dressing

1. Mix
    Juice of 1 lime
    1 teaspoon unpasteurized honey
    ¼ teaspoon gray sea salt
    Tahini to taste

Umeboshi Dressing

1. Mix
4 to 6 tablespoons olive oil *
1 teaspoon honey *or* rice syrup
⅓ or ½ teaspoon umeboshi paste

2. Toss with salad

Garlic Dressing

1. Mix
Oil
3 crushed cloves of garlic
¼ teaspoon gray sea salt
¼ teaspoon stevia, if desired

Tofu Dip

1. Mix
¼ cup olive oil*
2 tablespoons rice vinegar
¼ teaspoon *Fines-herbes*
¼ cup mashed tofu

2. Serve with raw vegetables

---

* In salad dressings as in other dishes, always use cold, first-pressed oils.

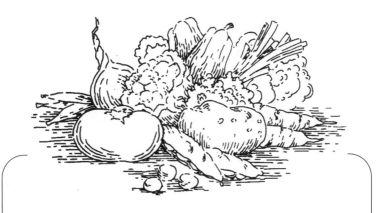

Vegetable Purées

Spinach Purée

1. Cook for 10 minutes
2 to 3 cups distilled water
½ cup chopped leek
¼ cup finely-chopped celery

2. Add the following ingredients and turn off heat
¼ cup chopped mushrooms
1 teaspoon salt-free instant powdered vegetable broth
4 cups spinach

3. Blend into a purée

4. Serve hot

Carrot Purée

1. Cook the following ingredients for 15 minutes
2 cups chopped carrots
½ cup chopped turnip
¼ cup sliced leek
3 or 4 cups water

2. Turn off heat and add
3 chopped mushrooms
½ teaspoon *Fines-herbes*
½ teaspoon salt-free instant powdered vegetable broth

3. Blend into a purée

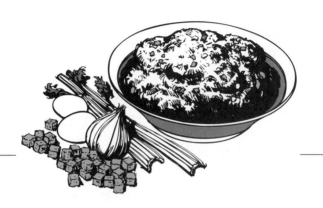

Pâtés and
Spreads

Hummus

1. Blend together

2 cups cooked chickpeas
2 cups water
¼ teaspoon *Fines-herbes*
Juice of one lime
2 tablespoons olive oil
Gray sea salt, if desired
1 teaspoon fennel seeds

2. Serve with bread for noontime meal or as a snack

Vegetable Pâté

1. Mix
3 cups finely-chopped carrots
½ cup ground sunflower seeds
½ cup brown rice flour
1 cup distilled water
1 teaspoon paprika

2. Mix separately
½ cup distilled water
1 or 2 teaspoons barley miso
1 tablespoon hatcho miso
½ teaspoon fennel seeds
3 tablespoons saffron oil

3. Mix all the ingredients together

4. Spread on a greased tray

5. Bake in oven at 175 °C (350 °F) for 30 minutes

Tofu Spread

1. Carefully mix
1 cup soft tofu, mashed
¼ cup cooked carrots, puréed
¼ cup minced parsley
¼ cup chopped onion

2. Prepare sauce by mixing
Lime juice
Honey *or* stevia
Sea salt to taste

3. Serve with bread or rice cakes

Avocado Tofu

1. Mash together
400gr mashed tofu
1 avocado
5 cloves of garlic, minced
1 green onion, minced
2 slices ginger
1 teaspoon vegetable salt
¼ cup water

2. Add and mix well
4 finely-chopped parsley sprigs
1 teaspoon paprika
Lime juice
1 tablespoon instant powdered vegetable soup, if desired

3. Serve as an hors-d'oeuvre or as a snack, with bread or rice cakes

Chicken or Veal Liver Pâté

1. Cook for 20 minutes
100gr chicken livers *or* veal liver, cut in pieces
50gr chopped veal
½ cup distilled water

2. Mash the above ingredients with
½ teaspoon citronella powder *or* fennel seeds
1 or 2 tablespoons crushed ginger
Vegetable *or* sea salt, if desired
½ teaspoon paprika

3. Sprinkle onto the pâté
½ teaspoon *Fines-herbes*

4. Bake in oven at 175 °C (350 °F) for 30 to 40 minutes

5. Serve with bread

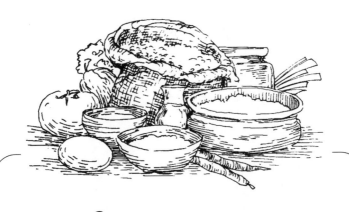

Noon and Evening Grains

General guidelines for cooking grains

1. Cook grains in distilled or spring water

2. Add vegetables:
Celery, carrots
and tofu, in pieces, *or* chicken

3. Season with
Tekka
Light tamari sauce
or gomashio sauce

Buckwheat

1. Cook for 30 minutes
2 or 3 cups water
1 cup raw buckwheat
1 tablespoon sunflower seeds

2. Serve with
Parsley
Olive oil
Garlic

Millet

1. Cook for 40 to 50 minutes
   1 cup millet
   1 tablespoon sunflower seeds
   3 cups water

2. Serve with fish, tofu, white meat

Quinoa

1. Cook for 30 minutes
   3 cups water
   1 cup quinoa
   1 tablespoon sunflower seeds

2. Serve with fish, tofu, white meat

Millet and Quinoa

1. Cook for 40 minutes
   3 cups water
   ½ cup quinoa
   ½ cup millet
   2 tablespoons sunflower seeds

2. Serve with fish, tofu, white meat

Quinoa and Arrow-root

1. Cook for 30 minutes
   3 cups water
   ½ cup arrow-root
   ½ cup quinoa
   2 tablespoons sunflower seeds

2. Serve with fish, tofu, white meat

Brown Rice

Note: If using wild rice, keep in mind that it requires more water and longer cooking time than brown rice.

1. Cook for 40 minutes
   1½ cups water
   1 cup brown rice
   1 tablespoon sunflower seeds

2. Serve with raw or cooked vegetables

Rice with Chicken and Mushrooms

1. Cook for 30 minutes
   1 cup brown rice
   1½ cups water

2. Add
   ½ cup sliced chicken
   4 soaked shiitake mushrooms, sliced
   or ¼ cup sliced white mushrooms
   2 tablespoons ginger slices

3. Continue cooking on low for 20 to 30 minutes longer

4. Add
   Light tamari sauce
   1 finely-chopped green onion

5. Serve hot with a salad

Paella

1. Cook in a frying pan for 20 to 30 minutes
½ cup sliced chicken breast
¼ cup thinly-sliced fresh lotus root
or daikon
½ cup distilled water *or* chicken broth
½ cup fresh peas

2. Add
2 or 3 cups brown rice, pre-cooked in chicken broth
1 chopped green onion
Light tamari *or* teriyaki sauce
½ cup sliced white mushrooms
¼ cup celery and carrots, thinly sliced

3. Continue cooking for 5 minutes

4. Serve hot with a salad

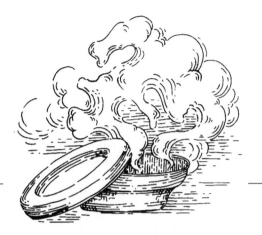

Stews

Vegetarian Stew

1. Cook for 30 minutes
1 cup tofu pieces
¼ cup soaked lotus root, thinly sliced
¼ cup soaked shiitake mushrooms, chopped
3 cups distilled water
Light tamari sauce *or* barley miso

2. Turn off heat and add
1 green onion, chopped

3. Serve hot with cooked whole grains

Tofu Ratatouille

1. Cook for 30 to 40 minutes
4 taro roots, peeled and cubed
½ cup tofu pieces (*or* chicken)
2 cups pumpkin pieces
5 cups distilled water
2 slices fresh (*or* dried and soaked) lotus root, chopped

2. Add
1 green onion, chopped
¼ teaspoon *Fines-herbes*
2 tablespoons light tamari sauce

3. Serve hot

Tofu and Tempeh Stew

1. Cook on medium heat for 15 to 20 minutes
½ cup soaked tofu
¼ cup tempeh pieces
¼ cup fresh lotus root (*or* daikon), sliced
¼ cup mushroom pieces (soaked reishi *or* white mushrooms)
3 or 4 cups distilled water

2. Add
Instant powdered vegetable *or* chicken broth
1 thinly-sliced green onion

3. Serve with rice

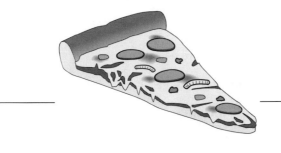

Pizzas

Pizza Dough

1. Mix
1 cup spelt flour
½ cup water
2 tablespoons saffron oil
1 tablespoon Soya margarine

2. Knead for 5 minutes

3. Let stand for 30 minutes

Tahini Pizza

1. Mix
¼ cup finely-chopped celery
1 cup finely-chopped sweet potato
½ cup finely-chopped carrots
¼ teaspoon gray sea salt
or 1 tablespoon salt-free instant powdered vegetable broth
Tahini, to taste

2. Stretch dough onto a greased cookie sheet

3. Spread ingredients over the dough

4. Sprinkle with Fines-herbes

5. Bake in oven at 175 °C (350 °F) for 20 to 30 minutes

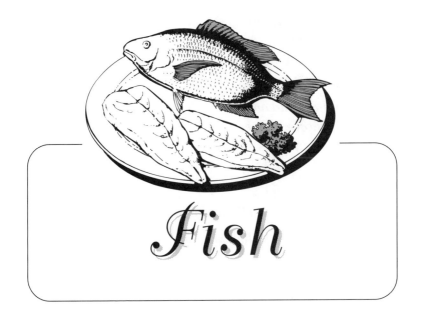

Fish

Steamed Fish

1. Steam for 30 minutes
1 fresh fish of your choice
½ cup chopped mushrooms
2 tablespoons crushed ginger

2. Turn off heat and add
1 green onion, chopped
Sesame *or* sunflower *or* olive oil

3. Serve with
Lettuce *or* watercress
Prepared fish sauce *or* light tamari sauce

4. Serve with rice or millet, according to taste

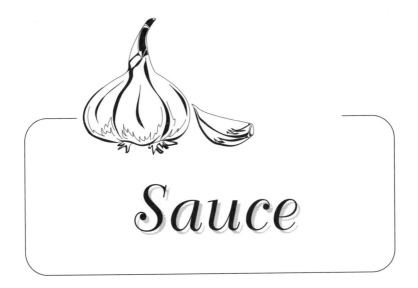

Sauce

Sweet-and-Sour Soya Sauce
(For grilled fish and imperial rolls)

1. Mix
Lime juice
4 or 5 tablespoons light tamari sauce
or fish sauce
1 cup distilled water
1 tablespoon honey
¼ teaspoon paprika
Cayenne pepper
2 crushed garlic cloves

2. Store in refrigerator

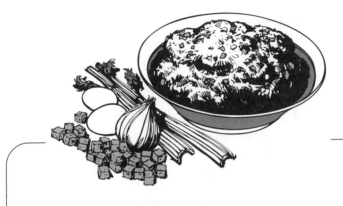

Soya

Soya Burger

1. Mix for 10 minutes
    ½ cup chickpea flour
    ½ cup Soya flour
    ⅓ cup sunflower and sesame seeds
    2 cups cooked sweet rice
    ¼ cup soaked dehydrated vegetables
    4 tablespoons light tamari sauce
    3 or 4 cups distilled water
    4 tablespoons safflower oil

2. Shape the mixture into a burger

3. Place on a pan rubbed with saffron oil

4. Bake in oven at 175 °C (350 °F) for 30 to 40 minutes

5. Serve on rye bread

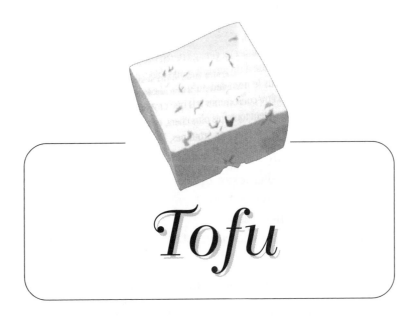

Tofu

Tofu is made from crushed Soya beans, cooked and set with magnesium chloride or calcium phosphate.

There are three kinds: hard and dry, firm, soft.

Note: In most recipes, tofu can be replaced with soaked tofuki (dried tofu).

Squash or Pumpkin Stuffed with Tofu

1. Hollow out
A medium-sized Chinese squash *or* buttercup pumpkin

2. Mix
3 to 5 white mushrooms *or* shiitake *or* soaked reishi, cut in pieces
1 finely-chopped green onion
1 cup mashed tofu
or ½ cup chopped chicken *or* veal
1 tablespoon arrow-root flour
½ teaspoon fennel seeds
Salt-free instant powdered vegetable broth *or* light tamari sauce

3. Put this mix into the squash or pumpkin

4. Boil with 4 to 6 cups distilled water for 30 minutes in a tightly covered saucepan

5. Serve hot with rice or millet

Double-boiler Tofu

1. Mix well in a bowl
2 cups hard tofu, mashed
4 tablespoons soaked dried vegetables
1 tablespoon nutritional yeast
1 tablespoon salt-free instant powdered vegetable broth
1 tablespoon arrow-root flour
Chopped green onion *or Fines-herbes*
¼ cup soaked transparent vermicelli cut in pieces

2. Cook in top half of a double boiler for 30 minutes

3. Serve hot with rice or other grains

Baked Tofu

1. Marinate for 2 hours
300gr tofu in thick slices
3 tablespoons light tamari sauce
¼ teaspoon *Fines-herbes*
1 tablespoon honey *or* ¼ teaspoon stevia
½ teaspoon paprika
½ teaspoon fennel seeds

2. Bake in oven at 175 °C (350 °F) for 30 to 40 minutes

Baked Tofu Sushi

1. Use
A bamboo mat to make sushi
Nori leaves
3 cups cooked whole-grain sweet rice
Umeboshi
Wasabi (green mustard)
Sliced baked tofu *or* sliced marinated salmon *or* sliced baked tempeh
Marinated ginger
Marinated carrot and daikon
Cucumber and celery, cut into strips
Sliced red pepper

2. Lay out nori on bamboo mat

3. Spread some rice over the nori and a bit of umeboshi and wasabi over the rice

4. Add vegetables and tofu (or salmon or tempeh)

5. Roll up

6. Cut into slices and serve

Ginger Tofu

1. Cook for 10 minutes
½ cup water
200gr sliced soft tofu
¼ cup ginger, cut into strips
¼ cup soaked reishi mushrooms *or* white mushrooms, cut in pieces
Light tamari sauce
¼ cup dried lily flowers, if desired

2. Add
1 green onion, chopped

3. Serve with rice or other grains

Curried Tofu

1. Cook for 20 minutes
300gr soft tofu, cubed
2 cups distilled water
½ cup carrot, cut into pieces
5 mushrooms, cut into pieces
1 teaspoon paprika
¼ teaspoon turmeric
3 grains star-anise
½ teaspoon fennel seeds *or* citronella
Gray sea salt *or* vegetable salt

2. Serve with rice

Tofu with Carrots

1. Mix

½ cup grated carrot

½ cup mashed soft tofu

2 or 3 white mushrooms *or* soaked and chopped reishi (black fungus)

1 teaspoon salt-free instant powdered vegetable broth

1 green onion, chopped

1 tablespoon arrow-root flour

2. Roll paste into little balls and place them in a steamer

3. Steam for 30 minutes

4. Serve hot with rice or other grains and light tamari sauce

Tofu with Onions

1. Cook for 10 to 20 minutes
½ carrot, cut into small pieces
3 slices finely-chopped ginger
1 cup soft tofu
3 soaked shiitake mushrooms, chopped
or ¼ soaked Kombu leaf, chopped
2 tablespoons light tamari sauce
½ cup distilled water

2. Add
½ onion, chopped
1 tablespoon sesame oil
¼ teaspoon *Fines-herbes or* ½ teaspoon fennel seeds

3. Serve hot

Tofu with Burdock

1. Heat for 10 minutes
½ cup soft tofu, in pieces
½ cup thinly-sliced carrot and burdock
3 soaked shiitake mushrooms *or* white mushrooms,
in pieces

2. Turn off heat and add
2 tablespoons sunflower *or* sesame *or* Soya oil
Light tamari sauce

3. Serve with rice or other grains

Tofu with Lotus Root

1. Heat for 10 to 20 minutes

¼ cup soft tofu *or* chicken in pieces

¼ cup fresh lotus root (*or* dried and soaked) cut into thin slices

½ cup distilled water

3 white mushrooms *or* soaked shiitake, cut in thin slices

¼ cup thinly-sliced carrot

2. Add the following ingredients and turn off heat

Sesame *or* sunflower *or* olive oil

2 tablespoons sliced almonds

Light tamari sauce

Coriander *or* parsley

3. Serve hot with rice or millet

Tofu with Mushrooms

1. Mix
200gr sliced soft tofu
¼ cup shiitake *or* reishi (soaked) *or* white mushrooms,
chopped
5 slices ginger, crushed
¼ teaspoon paprika
3 tablespoons light tamari sauce
¼ teaspoon fennel seeds

2. Bake in oven at 175 °C (350 °F) for 30 minutes

3. Serve with rice or salad

Tofu with Mushrooms and Miso

1. Cook in double boiler for 30 minutes
3 quail eggs, cooked and shelled
1 cup soft tofu, in large cubes
¼ cup tofuki, in pieces
3 soaked shiitake mushrooms
5 slices ginger
½ cup daikon *or* carrot, chopped
1 teaspoon hatcho miso *or* rice miso
3 tablespoons light tamari sauce
¼ cup water

2. Add
Coriander and finely-chopped green onion

3. Serve with rice

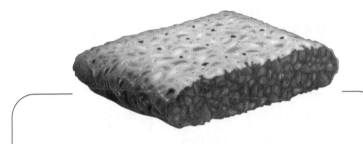

Seitan
and Tempeh

Seitan

1. Mix well
   1 cup gluten
   1 tablespoon paprika
   ¼ teaspoon ground ginger

2. Mix well
   1 tablespoon hatcho miso
   1 tablespoon natto miso
   4 or 5 cups lukewarm distilled water, to make a dough

3. Combine the above ingredients and mix thoroughly

4. Knead dough for several minutes

5. Let stand for 30 minutes

6. Cut the seitan into pieces

7. Boil in water for 30 to 40 minutes

8. Serve with sauce (see below)

Sauce

1. Mix
   1 soaked wakame strip, cut into pieces
   or ¼ cup soaked reishi mushrooms
   3 cups distilled water
   2 tablespoons mugi miso

2. Cook over medium heat for 10 minutes

Sautéed Seitan with Vegetables

1. Cook for 10 minutes
¼ cup seitan, cubed
½ cup distilled water
¼ cup sliced mushrooms

2. Add
1 cup cabbage *or* Chinese squash (nappa or bok choy) *or*
Chinese broccoli, in pieces
½ carrot *or* ½ celery stalk, in thick slices
Light tamari sauce *or* hatcho miso

3. Continue cooking for another 5 minutes

4. Turn off heat

5. Add
3 tablespoons sliced almonds, if desired
1 tablespoon sesame oil

6. Serve hot with rice or other grains

Seitan with Seaweed and Mushrooms

1. Cook for 30 minutes
2 cups water
½ piece of soaked Kombu, thinly sliced
5 soaked shiitake mushrooms, thinly sliced
1 cup seitan, cubed
Light tamari sauce *or* hatcho miso, to taste
½ teaspoon fennel seeds

2. Add
2 tablespoons sesame oil

3. Turn off heat

4. Serve hot with rice or millet

Baked Tempeh with Ginger

1. Mix
1 cup tempeh, in small pieces
1 or 2 tablespoons honey *or* malt powder *or* ¼ teaspoon stevia
3 tablespoons chopped ginger
½ teaspoon paprika
Light tamari sauce *or* teriyaki sauce

2. Bake in oven at 175 °C (350 °F) for 30 minutes

3. Serve hot with cooked grains

Cookies

Oatmeal Cookies

1. Mix well

1 cup oats (oatmeal)
½ cup oat flour
1 or 2 tablespoons sunflower seeds
½ teaspoon stevia
or ¼ cup malt powder
1 cup distilled water

2. Make cookies 5 mm (¼ inch) thick

3. Bake in oven at 150 °C (300 °F) for 20 minutes

Sesame Cookies

1. Mix

2 cups spelt flour
¼ cup crushed sesame seeds
½ cup malt powder
¾ cup distilled water

2. Stir ingredients together and let stand for 5 minutes

3. Fold in

2 egg whites
2 tablespoons Soya margarine
1 teaspoon alum-free baking powder

4. Make cookies 5mm (¼ inch) thick

5. Sprinkle with sesame seeds

6. Bake in oven at 150 °C (300 °F) for 20 minutes

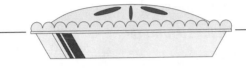

Pies

Pie Crust

1. Mix
2 cups spelt flour
1 cup distilled water
2 tablespoons Soya margarine
¼ teaspoon alum-free baking powder
2 tablespoons safflower oil

2. Knead dough for 10 minutes

3. Let stand for 30 minutes

Apple Pie

1. Mix
3 cups peeled, sliced apples
½ teaspoon ground cinnamon
¼ teaspoon crushed ginger
3 or 4 tablespoons malt powder

2. Arrange piecrust dough in a greased pieplate

3. Place the above ingredients in the piecrust

4. Decorate pie with apple slices

5. Bake in oven at 175 °C (350 °F) for 20 minutes

6. Cook for 10 minutes
¼ cup agar-agar, if desired
1 cup water

7. Baste pie with the liquid to obtain a jelly glaze

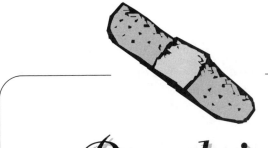

Poultice

To relieve pain in cancer patients, a ginger poultice can be beneficial.

1. Peel and grate
7.5 cm (3 inches) fresh ginger

2. Spread the warmed ginger directly onto the painful area and leave on for two minutes

3. Peel and grate 6 raw taros

4. Apply (immediately after the ginger poultice) directly onto the painful area and cover with a clean towel. Leave on for 30 minutes to one hour.

Repeat this operation twice a day for one month.

In the case of cysts or tumors, other poultices can be used, such as ones made with: clay, cabbage, mustard, castor oil, wheat germ, violet leaves.

Bibliography

●●●●●●●●●●●●●●●●●●●●●

The following books deal with the influence of nutrition on the development of specific diseases.

AIROLA, Paavo, Ph.D., 1974, 1995: *How to Get Well*, Health-Plus Publishers.

HONG-YEN, Hsu, oriental Ph.D., 1982: *Treating Cancer with Chinese Herbs*, Oriental Healing Arts Institute.

JANET, Jacques, M.D., *Préservez-vous du cancer*, Éditions Bionat.

LEDERER, Jean, M.D., 1986: *Alimentation et cancer*, Éditions Nauwelaerts-Maloine Éditeur.

About the Author

Bach-Tuyet is known in the French-speaking community as Blanche-Neige (Snow White in English). She was born in Vietnam to a family of doctors who practiced traditional Indochinese medicine.

She completed her studies in western medicine in Vietnam. She later studied public hygiene and international health statistics at the Université de Montréal. She has also worked in epidemiology at the Vietnam Health Ministry in collaboration with the World Health Organization (WHO), the United Nations International Children's Education Fund (UNICEF), and the United States Overseas Missions (USOM). Her extensive work has helped her understand and appreciate the correlation between the eating habits in various countries and the incidence of certain diseases.

This understanding led her to undertake extensive research on the impact nutrition has on the state and maintenance of health. She has lived in Montreal since 1969, where she pursues her research and provides counseling on nutrition and health.

The recipes in this book reflect her great experience in these areas. They are intended for those who care about the quality of their diet and its effects upon their health.

Acknowledgements

. . . .

I wish to thank my friend Michèle Juban, as well as my daughter Sophie Royer, for their assistance in proofreading this work.

I also want to thank my publisher Karole Lauzier, as well as Jacques Lalanne, for their editorial help. Finally, I thank Rémy Marcoux and Louis-Philippe Hébert, who strongly encouraged me to write this book.